THE COMPLETE MRCP

Photogra
Interpret
Questions
MRCP Part 2

D0230661

For Churchill Livingstone:

Publisher: Laurence Hunter
Project Editor: Barbara Simmons
Copy-editor: Ruth Swan
Project controller: Nancy Arnott
Design direction: Erik Bigland

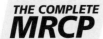

Photographic Interpretation Questions

MRCP Part 2

H L C Beynon BSc MD MRCP
Consultant Physician
Department of Rheumatology
Royal Free Hospital
London

J B van den Bogaerde MBChB PhD (Cantab) FCP(SA) MMed Int MRCP
Professor of Physiology
University of Pretoria
South Africa;
Reader in Physiology
St Mark's Hospital
Harrow

K A Davies MA MD FRCP
Senior Lecturer and Honorary Consultant
Department of Medicine
Imperial School of Medicine at the Hammersmith Hospital
London

Foreword by

Mark J Walport MA PhD FRCP FRCPath
Professor of Medicine, Chairman of the Division of Medicine, Imperial College
School of Medicine and Hammersmith Hospital, London

SECOND EDITION

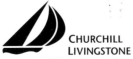

CHURCHILL
LIVINGSTONE

EDINBURGH LONDON NEW YORK PHILADELPHIA SAN FRANCISCO SYDNEY
TORONTO 1998

CHURCHILL LIVINSTONE
A Division of Harcourt Brace and Company Limited

Churchill Livingstone, 1-3 Baxter's Place, Leith Walk, Edinburgh EH1 3AF

© Longman Group Limited 1991
© Churchill Livingstone, a division of Harcourt Brace and Company Limited 1998

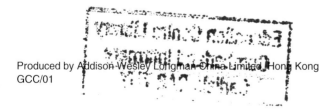 is a registered trademark of Harcourt Brace and Company Limited.

First edition 1991
Second edition 1998

ISBN 0443 056900

British Library of Cataloguing in Publication Data
A catalogue record for this book is available from the British Library.

Library of Congress Cataloging in Publication Data
A catalog record for this book is available from the Library of Congress.

Medical knowledge is constantly changing. As information becomes available,
changes in treatment, procedures, equipment and the use of drugs become
necessary. The author and publisher have, as far as it is possible, taken care to
ensure that the information given in the text is accurate and up-to-date.
However, readers are strongly advised to confirm that the information,
especially with regard to drug usage, complies with current legislation and
standard of practice.

Produced by Addison Wesley Longman China Limited, Hong Kong
GCC/01

Foreword to The Complete MRCP

The MRCP examination aims to test a broad range of clinical skills and background knowledge at an early stage of training in general medicine. The Part 1 examination provides an assessment of general medical knowledge and the written Part 2 assesses the ability to interpret clinical data and to identify those physical signs that can readily be photographed.

The format of the examination is influenced by the large number of candidates and the necessity to provide a test of uniform standard. Multiple choice questions (MCQs) provide a standardised assessment of knowledge. Studies conducted in disciplines other than medicine have shown that MCQs provide a discriminator of abilities that correlates with other tests such as the writing of essays. Animated discussion of the answers to multiple choice questions posed in the examination often engenders paranoia about the ambiguity or idiocy of particular questions. In reality, the answers to clinical questions are rarely black and white, as demanded by MCQs. However, the occasional obscure or ambiguous question that slips into the exam will be detected during marking of the papers and will not be used again. Such questions will only damage individual candidates if the fury they engender at the time disturbs a balanced approach to answering the remainder of the questions. The 'grey' cases and photographic questions provide tests that approximate more closely to the reality of the bedside and probe comprehension of relevant clinical physiology and pathology.

This series of three books has been written by a team of physicians who have not yet forgotten the agonies of the MRCP examination and who participate actively in teaching others who are about to confront the same hurdle. These books provide stimulating examples of the types of question encountered in all three sections of the MRCP examination, and provide an entertaining and informative journey through many of the highways and byways of medicine

London 1998   M.J.W.

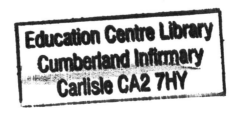

Preface

This is the third book in the series 'The Complete MRCP' and is
complementary to books 1 and 2. Book 1 contains 300 MCQs with
expanded answers and covers Part 1 of the MRCP. Books 2 and 3
cover the photographic material and the data and grey case section
of Part 2 of the MRCP exam.

During the photographic interpretation section 20 photographs
covering the physical signs, radiology, haematology, microbiology
and histopathoiogy are presented and the candidate has 40 minutes
to answer the accompanying questions. Each photograph is usually
accompanied by some relevant history which helps the candidate
make the most appropriate diagnosis. The material presented here is
representative of that shown in the exam and the expanded answers
should facilitate revision.

We hope this series will be both stimulating and helpful for
candidates preparing for the examination.

We gratefully acknowledge the contributions of Dr C Marguerie
and Dr C Craddock to the first edition of this book.

1998
H.L.C. Beynon
J.B. van den Bogaerde
K.A. Davies

Acknowledgements

We would like to thank Professor M J Walport for all his support and advice throughout the preparation of the manuscript. We are also grateful to the following people for contributing clinical material: Dr R W A Jones, Dr P Nihoyannopoulos, Professor M J Walport, Dr A K So, Dr A J Rees, Dr A C Chu, Professor G F Joplin, Dr H Montgomery, Dr A Zumla, Mr R J Morries and Professor E M Kohner.

This lady presented with hypertension and proteinuria.
a) What physical sign is present?
b) What is the diagnosis?

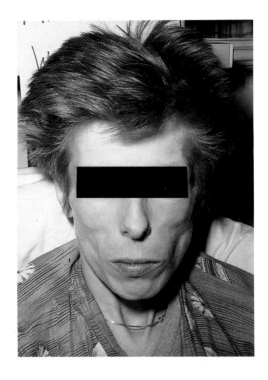

a) Facial lipodystrophy — there is marked loss of subcutaneous tissue around the face.
b) The patient has a mesangiocapillary glomerulonephritis Type 2.

Two types of mesangiocapillary (membranoproliferative) glomerulonephritis are recognized; both have mesangial cell proliferation, diffuse thickening of the glomerular capillary walls and, on electron microscopy, electron dense deposits in the capillary basement membrane. Type 1 has subendothelial deposits; Type 2 is characterized by intramembranous deposits of electron dense material (dense deposit disease).

In Type 2 mesangiocapillary glomerulonephritis C3 is found along capillary loops but unlike Type 1 no immunoglobulins are found. An autoantibody, the C3 nephritic factor, is found in 70% of Type 2 mesangiocapillary glomerulonephritis; this stabilizes C3bBb (the alternative complement pathway convertase enzyme) allowing uncontrolled activation of the alternative pathway leading to low serum levels of C3, factor B and properdin but normal C4. There is a well recognized association between Type 2 mesangiocapillary glomerulonephritis and partial lipodystrophy.

Mesangiocapillary glomerulonephritis usually presents as a nephritic or nephrotic illness. The natural history is one of a gradual deterioration to end stage renal failure over a 10 year period.

Question 2

This 58-year-old lady was previously well, and presented with a rash of 2 weeks duration. She also had 2^+ proteinuria.
a) What is the diagnosis?
b) What is her prognosis, and what treatment could you suggest?

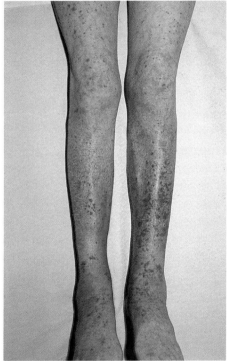

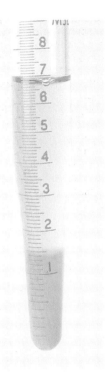

A
B

4 Answer to question 2

a) Slide A shows an extensive purpuric rash, and slide B shows an unspun cryoprecipitate. This lady has mixed cryoglobulinaemia, presenting with a vasculitic rash and glomerulonephritis.

b) It has recently become apparent that the majority of patients with mixed essential cryoglobulinaemia have underlying chronic hepatitis C infection. Alpha-interferon therapy has been shown to be effective in reducing cryoglobulin levels in patients with hepatitis C and concomitant cryoglobulinaemia. Patients with underlying renal disease have a worse prognosis than patients presenting with rash or arthralgias. Prognosis will also be affected by her underlying disease. Patients with renal disease may also benefit from plasma exchange, high dose steroids, or cyclophosphamide therapy.

Mesangiocapillary nephritis is the commonest type of glomerulonephritis seen in patients with essential mixed cryoglobulinaemia. Other clinical signs are a purpuric rash, usually leukocytoclastic, Raynaud's phenomenon, cutaneous ulcers or arthralgia. Sometimes pericarditis, thyroiditis or cold urticaria is seen, and mononeuritis multiplex may occur.

a) What is the abnormality? Give a differential diagnosis.
b) What is the likely underlying diagnosis in this 20-year-old man who has a high arched palate, bilateral pes cavus and kyphoscoliosis? List the other clinical signs you would look for to confirm your diagnosis.

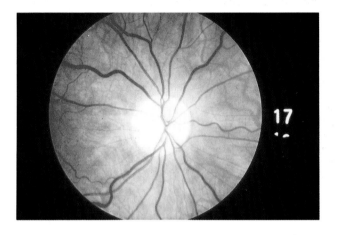

a) Optic atrophy — the disc is well demarcated and pale. Causes of optic atrophy include:

1. Acquired:
   - Glaucoma
   - Ischaemia: retinal artery occlusion
   - Demyelination: multiple sclerosis, giant cellarteritis
   - Infective choroidoretinitis: syphilis, toxoplasmosis
   - Retinal degenerative disease: retinitis pigmentosa
   - Trauma or pressure on the optic nerve: pituitary tumours, Paget's disease
   - Chronic papilloedema
   - Metabolic causes: diabetes, B_{12} deficiency
   - Toxic causes: lead, methyl alcohol, cyanide, tobacco–alcohol amblyopia.
2. Hereditary causes:
   - Leber's optic atrophy — commoner in males; there is uniocular visual loss in the second or third decade which eventually becomes bilateral
   - Friedreich's ataxia
   - DIDMOAD syndrome — **D**iabetes **I**nsipidus, **D**iabetes **M**ellitus, **O**ptic **A**trophy and **D**eafness (autosomal recessive).

b) The combination of optic atrophy, bilateral pes cavus, high arched palate and kyphoscoliosis suggests a diagnosis of Friedreich's ataxia. Friedreich's ataxia is characterized by spinocerebellar degeneration. The disease is inherited in an autosomal recessive manner normally, but occasionally the trait is dominant. Symptoms begin between the ages of 8 and 16 years. Neurological signs include:

1. Cerebellar signs — ataxia, dysarthria, nystagmus
2. Dorsal column loss
3. Peripheral neuropathy — absent reflexes
4. Corticospinal tract involvement — extensor plantar responses.

Cardiomyopathy and diabetes mellitus are also commonly found.

Question 4

a) What is the diagnosis?
b) What are the recognized pulmonary complications?

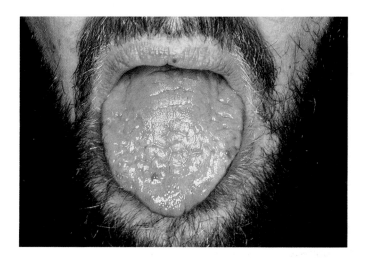

a) Hereditary haemorrhagic telangiectasia (Osler–Rendu–Weber syndrome).
The slide shows the typical telangiectatic lesions which are commonly seen in the nose and oral cavity. A telangiectasia is an enduring dilatation of small blood vessels, usually less than 1 mm in length. The disease is inherited in an autosomal dominant fashion although up to 20% of cases occur spontaneously.

Telangiectasia may be widespread throughout the body. The disease often presents in adolescence with an iron deficiency anaemia due to bleeding telangiectatic lesions in the gastrointestinal tract or nasal mucosa.

b) Pulmonary manifestations include:

1. Multiple coin lesions on the chest X-ray
2. Haemoptysis
3. Poor exercise tolerance because of right to left shunts.

Large pulmonary haemangiomas may be treated by embolization. Anecdotally, oestrogen therapy appears to decrease the frequency of bleeds, however no controlled trials have been undertaken.

a) What is the diagnosis in this 24-year-old African man?
b) Outline the recognized clinical features.
c) What are the recommended chemotherapeutic agents?

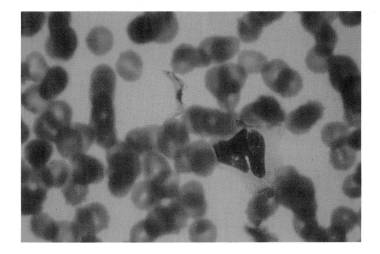

a) African trypanosomiasis. The slide shows an elongated trypanosome with its characteristic undulated membrane, anterior flagellum, prominent nucleus and darkly staining kinetoplast.

b) African trypanosomiasis occurs in two forms:

1. West African or Gambian sleeping sickness is caused by infection with *Trypanosoma brucei gambiense*.
2. East African or Rhodesian sleeping sickness is caused by infection with *Trypanosoma brucei rhodesiense*.

West African sleeping sickness is primarily a human infection whilst East African sleeping sickness is a zoonosis. Both types are spread by the tsetse fly.

1. Gambian sleeping sickness. Two to six weeks after a tsetse fly bite, a localized chancre develops. Several weeks later systemic trypanosomiasis develops. The patient has fever, malaise, cervical lymphadenopathy and splenomegaly. After a variable period of time the fever subsides, the lymphadenopathy regresses and the patient becomes asymptomatic. During this asymptomatic period invasion of the central nervous system occurs. Clinical features include a change in personality, daytime sleepiness, headache, backache, extrapyramidal signs and severe itching. Cardiac involvement is rare and mild. Finally patients become stuporous and die of secondary bacterial infections.
2. Rhodesian sleeping sickness is similar but the clinical course is more rapid; cardiac involvement is often severe and generally responsible for death. Haemolytic anaemia, thrombocytopenia, and disseminated intravascular coagulation are commoner in the Rhodesian form.

Serum IgM levels are raised in both types. Central nervous system involvement is associated with a lymphocytic CSF pleocytosis and a raised CSF IgM; trypanosomes are found in the CSF in 50% of cases.

The diagnosis is confirmed by identifying trypanosomes in the blood of early cases of Rhodesian sleeping sickness. Trypanosomes are less commonly found in the Gambian form so the diagnosis is made by gland puncture and aspiration.

c) Suramin is recommended for early stages of sleeping sickness but as it penetrates the CSF poorly, melarsoprol is used for late disease with central nervous system involvement.

This 24-year-old female has complained of a troublesome rash for the last 3 years.
a) What is the likely diagnosis?
b) Name three other conditions which can give this appearance.
c) What diagnostic tests would you consider?
d) What advice and drugs will be useful?

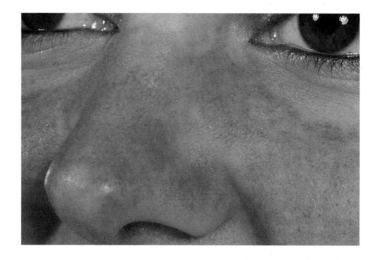

a) Photosensitive rash in a patient with cutaneous SLE.
b) Rosacea, lupus pernio, polymorphic light eruption, and acne may appear similar.
c) Antibodies against double stranded DNA and complement levels. Other tests include antibodies to extractable nuclear antigen (Sm, RNP, Ro, La), and antibodies against C1q. A high ESR and normal CRP would also support the diagnosis. A skin biopsy of non-lesional, non-light exposed skin will often demonstrate deposition of immunoglobulin and complement at the dermo-epidermal junction — this is a positive lupus band test. Urinalysis for underlying renal involvement is also needed.
d) For cutaneous lupus the patient should be told to avoid direct sunlight and to apply high factor suncreams which reflect back ultraviolet A and B radiation. Hydroxychloroquine or dapsone are used in severe cutaneous lupus. Recent data have shown that thalidomide is also useful in these patients. This drug must be used with circumspection in females of child bearing age. Thalidomide can also give a dose dependent sensory and motor neuropathy.

SLE is associated with many mucocutaneous features. The most characteristic are the photosensitive malar rash and discoid lupus. Subacute cutaneous lupus produces a generalized non-scarring rash which is either psoriasiform or annular. Bullous lesions, urticaria, angio-oedematous areas, a small vessel vasculitis (splinter haemorrhages), livedo reticularis (anti-phospholipid antibody positive, or cryoglobulin associated), lupus profundus (inflammation of subcutaneous fat), or Raynaud's phenomenon are seen. Mucosal ulcers may be deep and become infected with candida.

a) What is the cause of this appearance?
b) What is the differential diagnosis?
c) How would you establish a diagnosis?

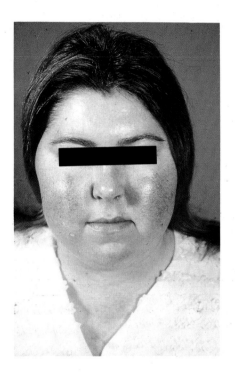

a) The slide shows the typical Cushingoid appearance with moon face and plethora. Other clinical features of Cushing's syndrome include: truncal obesity; hirsutism; easy bruising; osteoporosis; proximal myopathy; hypertension; diabetes; and depressive psychosis.

b) Cushing's syndrome is defined as the signs and symptoms of excess circulating levels of cortisol.
Differential diagnosis of Cushing's syndrome:

- Iatrogenic. Exogenous glucocorticoids are the commonest cause.
- Non-iatrogenic:

   1. ACTH dependent
      — Cushing's disease (80%): pituitary dependent bilateral adrenal hyperplasia, often the result of a basophil microadenoma
      — Ectopic ACTH from a benign or malignant tumour (5–10%), e.g. oat cell carcinoma, pancreatic tumour (hypokalaemic alkalosis, muscle weakness, hypertension, diabetes and increased skin pigmentation often prominent).
   2. ACTH independent
      — Primary adrenal adenoma (5–10%)
      — Primary adrenal carcinoma (rare, often associated with virilization)
      — Micronodular adrenal dysplasia (very rare)
      — Pseudo-Cushing's syndrome due to alcohol abuse or associated with a severe depressive psychosis.

c) Investigation of suspected Cushing's syndrome falls into two parts:

   1. Confirm cortisol excess:
      — Raised 24 hour free urinary cortisol.
      — Loss of diurnal variation in plasma cortisol concentration. However stress, pregnancy and the oral contraceptive pill may all raise the midnight cortisol and 24 hour excretion.
      — Failure of cortisol levels to suppress following administration of low dose dexamethasone (0.5 mg dexamethasone six hourly for 24 hours). However some normal, obese, depressed or alcoholic patients suppress poorly; patients with cyclical Cushing's may suppress normally.
   2. Determining the cause:
      — Plasma ACTH levels: very high in ectopic ACTH production; raised in Cushing's disease; undetectable with adrenal carcinoma and adenoma.
      — The high dose dexamethasone test suppresses ACTH and plasma cortisol in Cushing's disease (pituitary dependent).
      — Metyrapone test — metyrapone inhibits 11β hydroxylase and therefore cortisol synthesis and will cause a further rise in ACTH and thus 17-oxogenic steroids in Cushing's disease but not with ectopic ACTH.
      — Radiology. Skull X-rays. MRI scans of the pituitary and CT scans of the adrenal glands. Selenium-75 cholesterol scans for adrenal adenomas. Arteriography and venography to localize the exact source of ACTH.

This 10-year-old girl presented with a history of recurrent pyogenic infections, and tender painful gums. She had a marked peripheral blood polymorphonuclear leukocytosis, and normal lymphocyte count and immunoglobulin levels.

a) What is the most likely diagnosis?
b) How would you confirm the diagnosis?
c) What is the treatment and prognosis of this disorder?

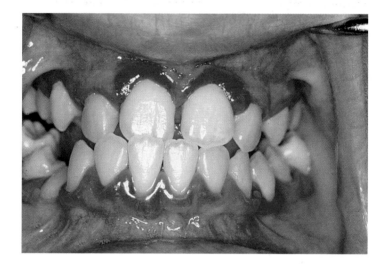

a) The history of recurrent infections and sore gums, in concert with a leukocytosis, raises the possibility of leukocyte adhesion molecule deficiency.

b) You would send her blood to a specialist centre where monoclonal antibody analysis of her peripheral blood cells would demonstrate an absence or reduction of the three β2 integrin molecules, LFA-1, CR3 and CR4.

c) After confirming the diagnosis treatment is supportive with antibiotic therapy and careful monitoring during acute infections. The definitive treatment is bone marrow transplantation. This has been performed successfully mostly by a group in France. Unfortunately donors are found in only about a third of patients. In patients with severe deficiency death in infancy is usual. Moderate deficiency results in death, usually in the second or third decade of life. Gene therapy might be used in future for these patients.

This patient died of a pneumonia. Post mortem investigation of her lungs demonstrated that although the lungs were filled with leukocytes, and particularly neutrophils, there was no migration of the neutrophils into the alveolar spaces. The infection could thus not be cleared in spite of antibiotic therapy, and the patient died.

a) What is the diagnosis and what is the likely aetiology?
b) List the other recognized ocular complications of this condition.

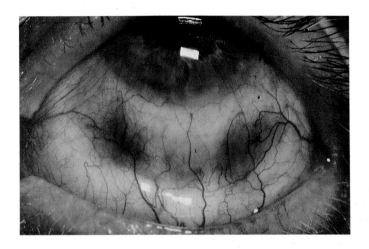

a) The slide shows scleromalacia perforans; 40% of these cases are associated with rheumatoid vasculitis. Scleritis with scleral thinning may also be seen with:

1. Systemic vasculitides, e.g. Wegener's granulomatosis and polyarteritis nodosa
2. Ankylosing spondylitis
3. Some infections, e.g. herpes zoster.

Scleritis is an ophthalmological emergency requiring high dose systemic steroids. Attacks of scleritis are usually painful and are always accompanied by episcleritis.

Scleritis may be classified anatomically into anterior and posterior types, and anterior scleritis may be further classified into diffuse, nodular and necrotizing varieties. Diffuse and nodular scleritis are typically painful and repeated attacks may lead to scleral thinning. Necrotizing scleritis is, however, often painless; breakdown of a scleral granuloma may leave a hole in the sclera — scleromalacia perforans. Vision is reduced in 40% of patients with scleritis due to the secondary complications of keratitis, uveitis, glaucoma, cataract and retinal detachment.

b) Whilst scleritis occurs in less than 1% of patients with rheumatoid arthritis, in general ocular involvement is common. 25% of patients with rheumatoid arthritis will have symptoms of keratoconjunctivitis sicca. Mild asymptomatic episcleritis is also common, self-limiting and is not related to disease activity. Other ocular complications include tenosynovitis of the ocular muscles, steroid-induced cataracts and chloroquine-induced retinopathy.

This 37-year-old woman presented acutely with a swollen, painful leg.
a) What two investigations are shown here, and what do they show?
b) How would you manage this patient?

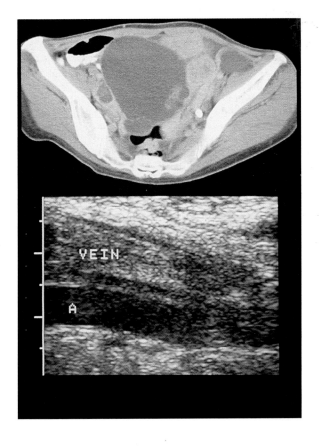

a) The examinations shown here are a pelvic CT scan and a Doppler ultrasound examination of the deep veins of the leg. A large ovarian mass is shown; this has caused a deep venous thrombus of the ipsilateral leg as a result of venous occlusion.

b) Anticoagulation is indicated, starting with intravenous heparin. Referral to a specialist gynaecological unit is indicated for histological diagnosis, which will determine future management.

An ovarian malignancy in a young patient suggests an underlying genetic abnormality. A thorough family history documenting maternal and female sibling malignancy is required. The BRCA 1 gene (breast cancer associated gene) and BRCA 2 gene are associated with ovarian and breast malignancy. Up to 85% of patients with mutations of this gene will develop breast cancer, while 60% will develop ovarian cancer. BRCA 2 gene mutations are also associated with breast and ovarian cancer, but linkage is weaker than the BRCA 1 gene. These genes are tumour suppressor genes, and more than 200 mutations have been defined. Environmental and dietary factors also affect the probability of developing malignancy.

This young woman presented with malaise and joint pains.
a) What investigation has been performed and what are the main abnormalities?
b) What is the likely diagnosis?

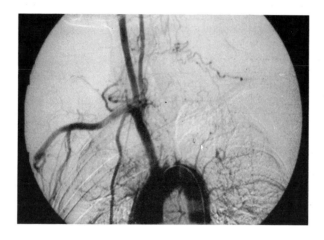

a) This is a digital subtraction arch aortogram which shows occlusion of the left common carotid and left subclavian arteries.
b) The diagnosis is Takayasu's arteritis. Despite occlusion of the left common carotid artery, cerebral perfusion is maintained via the circle of Willis.

Takayasu's arteritis typically presents in young women with malaise, early morning stiffness, polyarthralgia and/or polyarthritis. Histologically there is inflammation of the thoracic aorta and the proximal parts of its major branches. This may lead to absent pulses, an abnormal difference in the blood pressure between each arm, upper limb claudication, and hypertension if the renal arteries are involved.

Examination of the eye may reveal retinal haemorrhages, A–V fistula, and atrophy of the iris. Aortic valve disease is rare in Takayasu's arteritis. The ESR is usually raised.

Immunosuppressive treatment with corticosteroids and azathioprine or cyclophosphamide has improved the prognosis. Differential diagnosis of unequal limb pulses includes:

1. Giant cell arteritis
2. Syphilitic aortitis
3. Aortic dissection
4. Thrombosis
5. Buerger's disease
6. Abnormal vessel development.

This 30-year-old man receiving treatment for acute myeloid leukaemia complained of blurred vision.
a) Describe the abnormality present. What is the likely diagnosis?
b) How would you manage this problem?

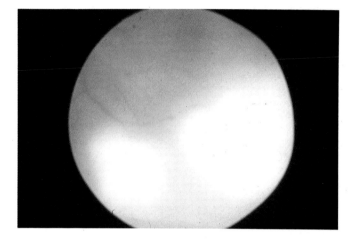

a) The slide shows white fluffy intravitreal ball-like lesions characteristic of *Candida* endophthalmitis. Fundal candidiasis may also manifest as yellow-white chorioretinal lesions or in chronic infections as white vitreoretinal scars often associated with traction. (Differential diagnosis — reactivation of toxoplasmosis.)

Disseminated candidiasis (*Candida albicans* and *Candida tropicalis*) occurs in patients who are immunosuppressed, debilitated, receiving parenteral nutrition, intravenous heroin abusers and who have received long courses of antibiotics.

b) The diagnosis of disseminated candidiasis is usually made clinically. Blood cultures are positive in only 50% of cases, however it is often possible to isolate candida from cutaneous lesions or bone marrow aspirates. Serological tests are of limited value in clinical management.

Combined treatment with amphotericin B and flucytosine is recommended for systemic candidiasis.

Question 13

This patient has had a barium enema.
a) List the abnormalities present on slide A and slide B.
b) What is the diagnosis?
c) Why does this patient have malabsorption?

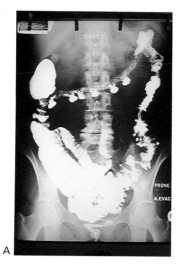

A

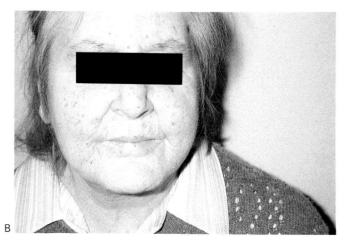

B

a) Slide A. Wide mouthed sacculations (pseudodiverticulae) and gall stones. Slide B. Multiple telangiectasia, skin tightening and beaking of the nose.

b) The patient has systemic sclerosis with the classical skin changes and gut involvement.

Other dermatological features include: sclerodactyly; Raynaud's phenomenon; calcification; pulp atrophy; ulceration; increased pigmentation; and vitiligo.

Systemic features include: pericarditis; myocardial fibrosis; pulmonary hypertension; pulmonary fibrosis; arthritis; polymyositis; and accelerated hypertension which can cause irreversible renal failure.

c) Scleroderma bowel malabsorption appears to be caused by stasis and bacterial overgrowth which causes a 'stagnant loop syndrome'.

Systemic sclerosis involves the bowel in over 50% of cases (histologically: smooth muscle atrophy; collagen deposition; fibrosis; and cholinergic denervation).

Gastrointestinal manifestations may be divided into six groups:

1. Microstomia and sicca syndrome
2. Oesophageal disease: abnormal peristalsis; dilatation of the proximal oesophagus; and distal strictures
3. Stomach and small bowel: bacterial overgrowth causing distension; colic; constipation; intermittent diarrhoea; and malabsorption
4. Colon: dilatation of the large bowel is often patchy, and results in characteristic sacculations seen above. Failure of peristalsis leads to pseudo-obstruction which may be fatal if perforation occurs
5. Pneumatosis intestinalis: benign, non-communicating, gas-containing cysts in the bowel wall
6. Associated autoimmune liver disease: chronic active hepatitis and primary biliary cirrhosis.

This young man presented with a 4 month history of a painful, swollen knee. The synovial biopsy is shown.
a) What is the diagnosis?
b) What other investigations would you perform?
c) How will you treat this patient?

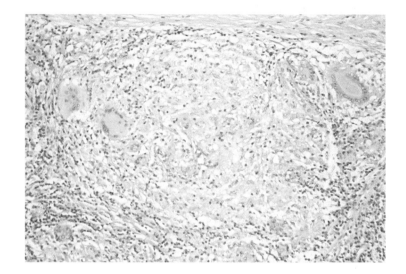

a) The biopsy shows a caseating granulomatous infiltrate of the synovium. Acid alcohol fast bacilli were seen on Ziehl–Neelsen stain. This patient has a tuberculous monarthritis.

b) FBC, ESR, biochemical profile, urinalysis, and chest X-ray are indicated. Joint aspiration with Ziehl–Neelsen or auramine staining is not sensitive, although it is specific. Synovial biopsy and culture is therefore imperative in patients with a chronic monarthritis in the absence of a firm diagnosis.

c) Therapy with a combination of drugs for at least 12 months.

Skeletal and joint tuberculosis in adults usually involves the thoracic spine, starting in the anterior body of the vertebra. In contrast to malignant destruction of the vertebral bodies, where the intervertebral discs are spared, infections lead to disc destruction. Only 50% per cent of patients have involvement of other organs, particularly the lung. The proximal femur, knee joints, and small hand joints are involved in descending frequency. Culture is 80% sensitive, and 100% specific, but may take up to 6 weeks.

a) List the abnormal physical signs.
b) What is the diagnosis?
c) How would you confirm your diagnosis?

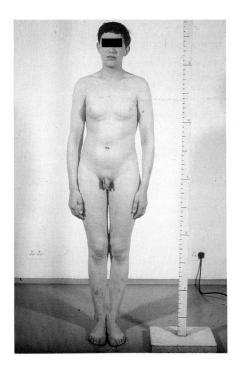

a) Gynaecomastia, small external genitalia, tall stature with eunuchoid proportions.

b) Klinefelter's syndrome (47 XXY).

The patients are hypogonadal, tall and thin, with small firm testes (seminiferous tubules and Leydig cells are abnormal) and high pitched voices. They are infertile although they can have erections and ejaculate; spermatozoa are never present. At puberty breasts develop, following which the diagnosis is usually made. Other features include: mental retardation, an increased risk of breast cancer and an increased risk of developing germ cell tumours.

c) Buccal smear cells from the buccal mucosa will be chromatin positive, i.e. there is a small darkly staining body (the Barr body) inside the nuclear membrane which is present in normal females but not in normal males. Its presence indicates there are two X chromosomes in the nucleus. The Lyon hypothesis states 'twelve days after fertilization one X chromosome in every cell of a female fetus becomes inactive, which of the two X chromosomes becomes inactive is decided at random'. The Barr body represents the condensed inactive X chromosome. Classically, patients with Klinefelter's have an XXY constitution caused by non-dysjunction in one parent.

A few cases are Barr body negative, and have some other chromosomal variation which will be revealed by chromosomal analysis. Rarely the syndrome is caused by congenital absence of germinal cells and is given the name del Castillo's disease.

This 25-year-old woman presented to the casualty department complaining of ankle pain.

a) What is the diagnosis?
b) List five recognized associations.
c) What is the single most important investigation to perform in casualty?

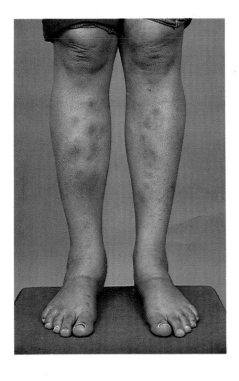

a) Erythema nodosum. The slide shows a swollen left ankle and
several red nodules over the extensor surfaces of the lower legs.
Erythema nodosum typically affects young adult females. Lesions are
red, raised, hot and tender. They erupt over a ten day period, usually
over the lower limbs, and may be accompanied by fever, malaise,
arthralgia and arthritis affecting the knees and ankles. In the second
week the erythema evolves into a blue-violet colour prior to healing.
A biopsy shows panniculitis with a perivascular mixed cell infiltrate.

b) The majority of cases are idiopathic but recognized associations
include:

1. Infections:
   — Streptococcal, Yersinia
   — Tuberculosis, leprosy
   — Psittacosis
   — Fungi: histoplasmosis, coccidioidomycosis, blastomycosis
   — Lymphogranuloma venereum, cat scratch fever,
2. Sarcoidosis
3. Drugs: sulphonamides; contraceptive pill; barbiturates;
   salicylates; and penicillins
4. Inflammatory bowel disease: ulcerative colitis, Crohn's disease,
5. Behcet's disease
6. Malignancy: lymphoma, leukaemia.

c) A chest X-ray should be performed to exclude sarcoidosis and
pulmonary tuberculosis.

Question 17

33

This 86-year-old lady presented with haematemesis due to a large gastric ulcer. A large effusion of her right shoulder was incidentally noted, and an X-ray performed. The patient admitted to sustaining an injury due to an accident with a supermarket trolley 6 months prior to presentation, resulting in chronic immobility of the joint.
a) What is the likely joint diagnosis?
b) What other investigations will confirm the diagnosis?

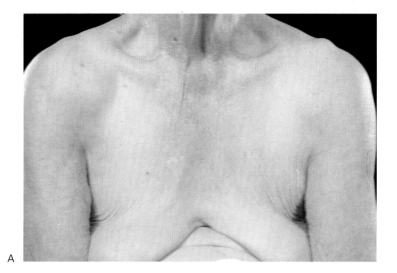

A

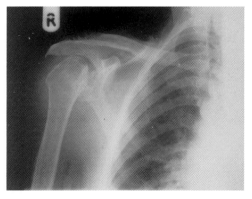

B

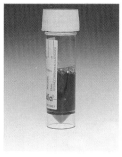

C

a) Milwaukee shoulder
b) — a large right shoulder effusion is clearly visible
— fluid aspirate was uniformly bloodstained, 200ml of such fluid was aspirated
— plain X-ray shows severe destruction of the humeral head. Alizarin red staining of the synovial fluid demonstrated hydoxyapatite crystals $(Ca_{10}(PO_4)6(OH)_2)$. Milwaukee shoulder often develops as a consequence of trauma and local degeneration of cartilage, resulting in deposition of hydroxyapatite crystals. This results in more destruction of the joint.

The ulcer in this patient was induced by high dose aspirin intake.

This peripheral blood film and X-ray belong to a 14-year-old boy who presented to casualty with pleuritic chest pain. What is the diagnosis?

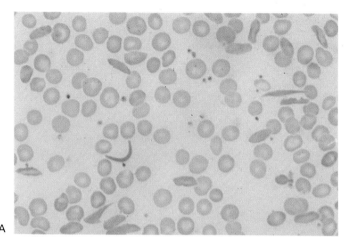

A

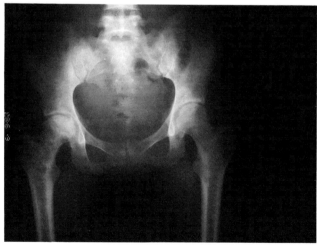

B

The peripheral blood film shows irreversibly sickled cells. There is avascular necrosis of the right femoral head on the X-ray. The diagnosis is sickle cell disease. This may be confirmed by haemoglobin electrophoresis.

Irreversibly sickled cells (crescenteric cells with two pointed extremities) are seen in sickle cell disease and Hb SC disease. Other features seen on the blood film of patients with sickle cell disease are target cells (although these are not as prominent as in Hb SC) and Howell–Jolly bodies caused by splenic infarction and consequent asplenism.

Recurrent small vessel thrombosis causes ischaemic damage to the femoral epiphyses and results in avascular necrosis of the femoral heads. X-rays show loss of joint space, collapse of the femoral head and sclerosis of the surrounding bone.

Avascular necrosis of the femoral head is more common in patients with high haematocrits and a long history of painful crises.

The pleuritic chest pain is a consequence of pulmonary vessel thrombosis.

a) What features does this X-ray show?
b) Give a differential diagnosis.

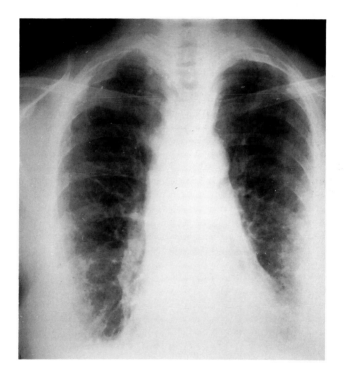

a) There is widespread interstitial shadowing with honeycomb changes present at both bases. These changes are characteristic of pulmonary fibrosis. There is marked dilatation of the central pulmonary arteries, with pruning of the peripheral vessles indicating pulmonary arterial hypertension.

b) The differential diagnosis of pulmonary fibrosis includes:

1. Cryptogenic fibrosing alveolitis — lower zones
2. Pneumoconiosis:
   - Coalworker's — upper and mid zones
   - Silicosis — upper zone
   - Asbestosis — lower zone (holly leaf pleural plaques)
   - Berylliosis — upper zone
3. Sarcoidosis — mid zone disease
4. Connective tissue diseases:
   - SLE ± high diaphragms
   - Scleroderma — lower zones
   - Rheumatoid arthritis ± nodules
   - Ankylosing spondylitis — upper zones
5. — Chronic extrinsic allergic alveolitis e.g. bird fancier's lung, farmer's lung — upper zones,
6. Drugs
   - Chronic high tension oxygen therapy
   - Nitrofurantoin
   - Amiodarone
   - Bleomycin
   - Busulphan
   - Melphalan
   - Chloramphenicol
   - Cyclophosphamide
7. Tuberculosis — upper zone fibrosis
8. Bronchopulmonary aspergillosis — upper zones
9. Previous irradiation — localized areas of fibrosis.

Rare causes of pulmonary fibrosis include:

- Histiocytosis X
- Lymphangiomyomatosis
- Tuberous sclerosis
- Neurofibromatosis.

This 30-year-old man recently returned from a holiday in the New Forest.

a) What is the diagnosis?
b) What are the other features of this disease?
c) How would you treat this man?

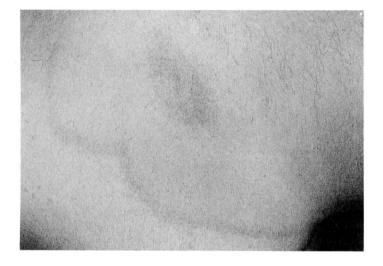

a) Lyme disease. The slide shows erythema chronicum migrans. The rash starts as red macules which spread, typically with central clearing, to form annular erythemas. Lyme disease is caused by the spirochete *Borrelia burgdorferi*; transmission is by ticks of the ixodes family, *Ixodes dammini* in the USA, *Ixodes ricinus* in Europe, whose natural hosts include horses, deer and field mice.

b) Lyme borreliosis may be divided into three stages.

Stage 1 (early infection):
Erythema chronicum migrans is the earliest feature in 70% of cases and one third remember the initial tick bite. Regional lymphadenopathy and mild fever may occur.

Stage 2:
Dissemination occurs days or weeks after the tick bite and is usually associated with fever and malaise. The other clinical features at this stage are diverse:

1. Skin: cutaneous annular lesions, diffuse erythema
2. Musculoskeletal system: arthralgia, myalgia
3. Nervous system: meningitis, radicular pain, cranial nerve palsies (a unilateral or bilateral VII nerve palsy is common), mononeuritis multiplex
4. Other manifestations include lymphadenopathy, atrioventricular block, pancarditis, conjunctivitis, mild hepatitis and microscopic haematuria.

Stage 3:
If the infection is left untreated many patients develop general fatigue and may develop late complications which include:

1. Skin rashes, acrodermatitis chronica atrophicans and lymphadenitis benigna cutis
2. Chronic arthritis (this is by far the commonest late complication occurring in up to 80% of untreated cases) and enthesopathy
3. Chronic encephalomyelitis, spastic paraparesis, cerebellar signs and dementia.

c) Oral tetracycline is the treatment of choice for Stage 1 borreliosis in adults; in children amoxycillin may be used.

This 37-year-old Afro-Caribbean woman with known SLE presented with an upper gastrointestinal haemorrhage, renal impairment and severe hypertension. The peripheral blood smear is shown.
a) What does the film show?
b) What other tests will you perform?
c) What is the diagnosis?
d) How would you manage this patient?

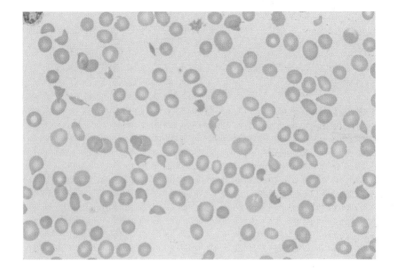

a) The slide shows anisocytosis, helmet cells, red cell fragmentation and thrombocytopenia.

b) Further tests are biochemical screen, ESR, complement levels, clotting screen, fibrin degradation products, lupus anticoagulant, and anticardiolipin levels.

c) The diagnosis is thrombotic microangiopathic haemolytic anaemia secondary to SLE.

d) Fresh frozen plasma infusion and plasma exchange, or high dose steroids are recommended. Plasma exchange is the most effective therapy.

Thrombotic microangiopathic haemolytic anaemia is often found in association with antibodies to CD36, a platelet glycoprotein. Anticardiolipin antibodies are found in some patients.

a) What is the clinical sign?
b) Give a differential diagnosis.

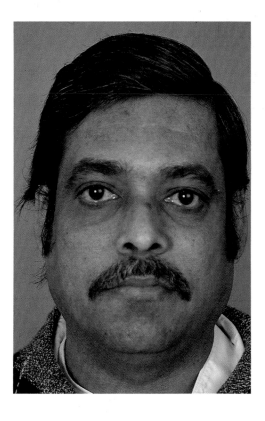

a) The patient has marked bilateral parotid swelling.
b) The differential diagnosis of bilateral parotid swelling includes:

1. Infections, e.g. mumps, bacterial parotitis
2. Sarcoidosis
3. Sjögren's syndrome
4. Cirrhosis (and high alcohol consumption per se)
5. Malignancy–lymphomas and parotid tumours
6. Cystic fibrosis
7. Diabetes
8. Amyloidosis/malnutrition
9. Malabsorption
10. Drugs, e.g. iodides, thiouracil, lead
11. Hyperlipidaemia
12. Acromegaly.

This is the blood film from a patient who presented with fever. The chest X-ray showed widespread shadowing.
a) What does the blood film show?
b) Give a differential diagnosis.

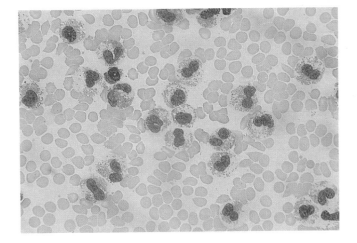

a) The blood film shows an increased number of eosinophils.
b) Pulmonary eosinophilia is defined as the combination of a peripheral blood eosinophilia with an eosinophilic lung infiltrate, usually manifest by shadowing on the chest X-ray.
Recognized causes of true pulmonary eosinophilia include:

1. Fungi: commonly *Aspergillus fumigatus*
2. Drugs and toxins, e.g. sulphonamides, tetracyclines, nitrofurantoin, non-steroidal anti-inflammatory drugs, Spanish toxic oil syndrome
3. Parasites: including ascaris, strongyloides, ankylostoma, filaria and schistosomiasis
4. Vasculitis, e.g. Churg–Strauss syndrome
5. Cryptogenic pulmonary eosinophilia: syndrome of fever, weight loss, eosinophilia and widespread peripheral alveolar shadowing. Asthma is common, rapid resolution in response to corticosteroids is the rule
6. Hypereosinophilic syndrome: very high eosinophil count 50 000–100 000/mm^2; it would appear to represent a myeloproliferative state.

High eosinophil counts without pulmonary involvement occur in eczema, scabies, pemphigus, pemphigoid, rheumatoid arthritis, Hodgkin's disease and Addison's disease.

This 23-year-old male presented with a dry cough and salivary gland swelling.
a) What investigation is shown here?
b) What is shown, and what is the diagnosis?
c) What other tests are useful?

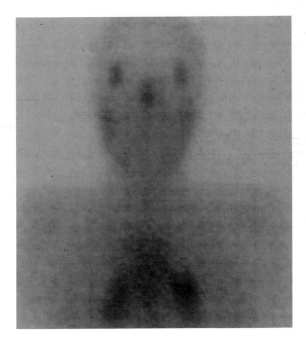

a) This is a gallium-67 scan.
b) Salivary, lacrimal and hilar glands show increased uptake, highly suggestive of sarcoidosis.
c) Chest X-ray may reveal hilar lymphadenopathy and a mid zone pulmonary infiltrate. Lung function tests may show a restrictive pattern with a low TLC. The serum ACE is increased in 70% of patients. Liver function tests may be abnormal and liver biopsy is positive for sarcoid granulomas in up to 80% of patients. The Kveim–Siltzbach test is still used in some centres. Fibre optic bronchoscopy with bronchial and transbronchial biopsy may reveal non caseating granulomas. Bronchoalveolar lavage typically shows an elevated lymphocyte count with an increase in the CD4 to CD8 ratio in sarcoidosis.
Serum immunoglobulins are often elevated. Hypercalcaemia and hypercalcuria are found in approximately 10% of patients. All patients suspected of having sarcoidosis should have a slit lamp examination performed to look for evidence of anterior uveitis. Non-caseating granulomas are typical, but do not differentiate between sarcoid or tuberculous granulomas, since 40% of tuberculous granulomas are non-caseating.

Question 25

a) What investigation has been performed?
b) What is the diagnosis?
c) What treatment would you prescribe?

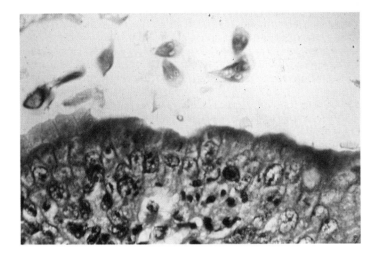

a) A small bowel biopsy.

b) Giardiasis with associated villous atrophy. *Giardia lamblia* is an anaerobic, flagellate parasite with two nuclei which infects the small bowel. It has a worldwide distribution (common in the tropics and endemic in Eastern Europe). The most important modes of transmission are food contaminated with cysts or inadequately treated water. Man to man spread is also recognized in homosexuals.

The incubation period is approximately two weeks. Giardiasis presents with anorexia, weight loss and acute or chronic diarrhoea with watery, yellow, foul smelling stools. The diagnosis is usually confirmed by finding faecal cysts. Alternatively, the trophozoites may be isolated from small bowel aspirates or be visible attached to the surface of epithelial cells in a small bowel biopsy. The amount of villous atrophy varies considerably, however a completely atrophic biopsy should raise the possibility of coeliac disease in addition to giardiasis. A small proportion of gluten-sensitive patients present when mild malabsorption is made worse by the additional insult of an intestinal infection. Malabsorption of fat, B_{12} and D-xylose is present in severe cases. Lactose intolerance may occur and persist for some time after treatment.

c) Treatment is with metronidazole or tinidazole. Symptoms should settle within 3–10 days.

This 65-year-old farmer presented to his GP with an enlarging lesion on his right arm.

a) What is the clinical diagnosis?

b) How would you manage him?

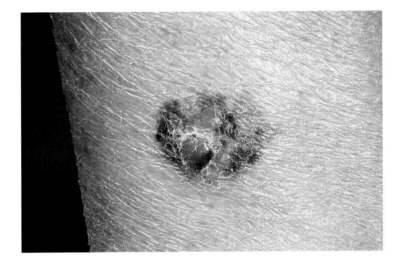

a) This slide shows the typical appearance of a malignant melanoma. An ill defined lesion, which exhibits nodularity, has variable colour and irregular margins.

b) This patient needs surgical referral, histological confirmation of the lesion, and excision. The lesion seen here is clearly a melanoma, but any suspicious lesion should be biopsied. Excision used to be disfiguring in the past, but recently a tumour depth of less than 1 mm would prompt a 1 cm margin, those deeper than 1 mm need a margin of 2 to 3 cm. Lymph node resection is not recommended for lesions of less than 1 mm, or more than 4 mm. For lesions with a depth of between 1 and 4 mm prophylactic lymph node excision is controversial. Chemotherapy is not helpful, and irradiation may be palliative. Experimental data has shown some role for immunotherapy with lymphokine activated killer cells.

Malignant melanoma has increased from a rate of 1/1000 in the 1950s to 1/100. Sunlight exposure produces a 2 to 4 fold increase of risk. Age and fair skin colour are risk factors, as is a positive family history. Caucasian patients have approximately 40 nevi at age 45, but more than 100 nevi are associated with increased risk. Large numbers of atypical nevi are associated with a lifetime risk in that individual of 10%.

The four types of melanoma are superficial spreading (80%), nodular (10–15%), lentigo maligna melanoma, and acral lentiginous. Prognosis is dependent on thickness of lesion and not type. A Breslow level of less than 0.75 mm has a 98% cure rate, 0.75–2 mm has a 30% mortality rate, while 4 mm or more has an 80% mortality. Even the thickest lesions have a cure rate of up to 10%.

This 45-year-old Caucasian woman drank a bottle of sparkling wine per day for 10 years. She presented to her GP with the rash shown below.
a) What clinical signs are seen here?
b) What is the likely diagnosis?
c) How would you manage this patient?

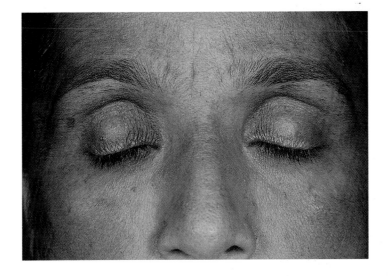

a) This patient has hyperpigmentation of her eyelids and forehead, with some scarring of her skin. This rash is typically found on sun exposed skin.

b) The diagnosis is porphyria cutanea tarda (PCT), which is familial, sporadic, or associated with toxins such as hexachlorobenzene. The enzyme defect is uroporphyrinogen decarboxylase, which is diagnosed in the familial form by testing the enzyme level in red blood cells. The toxic or sporadic form only shows the enzyme defect in the liver. Alcohol ingestion, intake of iron, or oestrogen exposure may precipitate this disease. Uroporphyrins and coproporphyrins are found in the urine, but uroporphyrin to coproporphyrin ratio is high in PCT.

c) This patient should stop drinking, and avoid sunlight. She should not take oestrogen-containing compounds. Phlebotomy is suggested, until 5–10 litres of venous blood have been taken off. If this is not tolerated chloroquine 250 mg three times a week may help.

PCT is the most common form of porphyria. It is more common in men, and patients are usually older than 35 years. Fatty liver is commonly seen, but cirrhosis is only found in 10% of patients. Neurological signs are not found, and cutaneous features include photosensitivity, blistering, pigmentation and depigmentation, hirsutism, scarring, thickening and milia.

This is the peripheral blood film from a previously fit 27-year-old woman who presents with tiredness and bruising.

a) What are the abnormalities present on the blood film and what is the diagnosis?

Treatment was started and four weeks later she developed fever, haemoptysis and shortness of breath

b) What complication has occurred (slide B)?

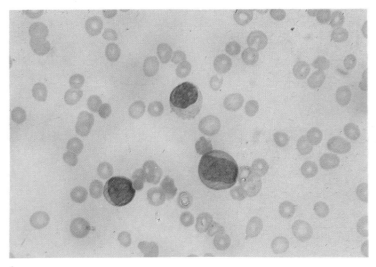

A

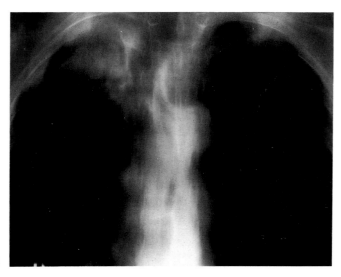

B

a) The peripheral blood shows large numbers of myeloblasts, and is from a patient with acute myeloid leukaemia. Myeloblasts are large cells with a high nuclear: cytoplasmic ratio and prominent nucleoli. They often contain Auer rods which, if present, are regarded as an indisputable marker of acute myeloid leukaemia.

b) The chest tomogram shows a large cavitating lesion in the right upper zone with a crescent sign characteristic of a mycetoma.

Aspergillus pneumonia is a frequent complication in immunocompromised patients, especially those with prolonged neutropenia. The diagnosis should be thought of in all susceptible patients and bronchoscopy with bronchoalveolar lavage performed early.

Intravenous amphotericin B is the treatment of choice. Flucytosine may be added for additional benefit.

This 25-year-old woman presented with a rash.
a) What is shown?
b) What are the possible causes of these lesions?

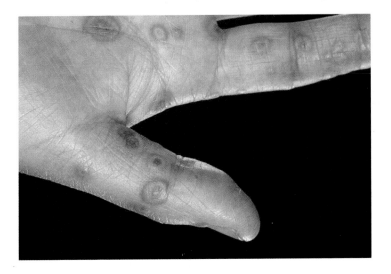

a) Erythema multiforme is shown, with typical target lesions.
b) Recognized causes include:
1. Idiopathic
2. Infections: herpes and mycoplasma are the most common; streptococci, typhoid, such as histoplasmosis, or orf are also associated
3. Drug: sulphonamides, barbiturates, sulphonylureas, salicylates and phenytoins
4. Systemic diseases such as SLE and ulcerative colitis
5. Carcinoma or lymphoma.

This patient had a mild form of erythema multiforme, but in its most severe form, the Stevens–Johnson syndrome, a widespread vasculitis is seen. Fever, conjunctivitis, corneal scarring, epidermal necrolysis, urethritis, glomerulonephritis and pneumonitis may be seen. High dose steroid and antibiotic therapy reduces mortality which is, however, still high.

This 40-year-old Nigerian man presented with bilateral foot drop. He had palpable common peroneal and supraorbital nerves.
a) What is the diagnosis?
b) How would you confirm your diagnosis?
c) What drugs may be used to treat this condition?

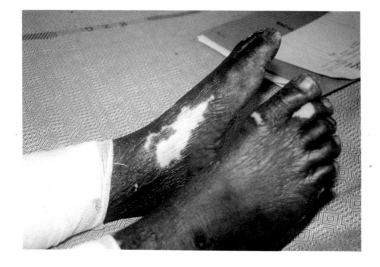

a) Tuberculoid leprosy: the combination of hypopigmented lesions and thickened peripheral nerves is typical of the tuberculoid spectrum of leprosy.
Leprosy is caused by the acid fast intracellular bacillus *Mycobacterium leprae*. The pattern of clinical disease is determined by the host's immune response. In tuberculoid lesions there is a strong cell-mediated response and *M. leprae* are rarely seen; in contrast the cell-mediated response is poor in lepromatous leprosy and bacilli are abundant. The lepromin skin test, a measure of cell-mediated immunity, is strongly positive in tuberculoid but is negative in lepromatous leprosy.
   Patients with tuberculoid leprosy usually have one to three cutaneous lesions. Typically these are large and annular, with a raised outer edge and a hypopigmented centre. Alternatively, as in this case, hypopigmented macules may occur. The tuberculoid skin lesions are classically anaesthetic, anhidrotic and have lost hair. Peripheral nerve enlargement is common, particularly in the borderline tuberculoid group.

b) Diagnosis is confirmed histologically. Tuberculoid lesions contain granulomas but almost no bacilli. Caseation is not a feature of tuberculoid skin granulomas but may be present in nerve lesions. The lepromin skin test is positive.

c) Patients should receive at least two chemotherapeutic agents, since resistance to dapsone is increasing. Currently the recommended treatment of tuberculoid (pauci-bacterial) leprosy is daily dapsone and monthly rifampicin for six months. Clofazimine, prothionamide and ethionamide have also been used.

Note: triple therapy with dapsone, rifampicin and clofazimine is recommended for lepromatous leprosy.

a) List the two physical signs.
b) Urine microscopy showed red blood cells and several red cell casts per high powered field. What is the diagnosis?
c) List the other recognized clinical features.
d) How should this man be treated?

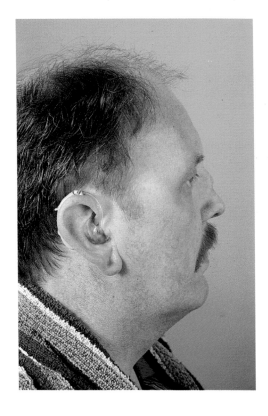

a) Collapsed nasal bridge and a right hearing aid.

b) The urine sediment indicates glomerulonephritis. The combination of upper respiratory tract disease (collapse of the nasal bridge and hearing loss) and glomerulonephritis strongly suggests a diagnosis of Wegener's granulomatosis.

c) Wegener's granulomatosis is a small vessel vasculitis which most commonly involves: the upper respiratory tract (involvement of nose, sinuses, ears); the lower respiratory tract (nodular and cavitating lesions); and the kidney (focal necrotizing glomerulonephritis). Evidence of disease in two or more of these sites with histology showing a small vessel necrotizing vasculitis, with associated granuloma formation, confirms the diagnosis. Anti-neutrophil cytoplasmic antibodies (ANCA) are sensitive serological markers for Wegener's granulomatosis and microscopic polyarteritis nodosa (a related small vessel vasculitic illness). Patients with Wegener's are usually C-AMCA positive, the antibodies being directed against proteinase 3.
Other clinical features include:

1. Fever and malaise
2. Polyarthralgia
3. Skin lesions: a vasculitic rash, nail fold infarcts
4. Eye lesions: scleritis, uveitis, proptosis
5. Cardiac lesions: pericarditis, myocarditis, arrhythmias
6. Neurological lesions: mononeuritis multiplex, intracerebral granulomas.

d) Before effective treatment was available, 80% of patients with Wegener's granulomatosis died within one year, and the mean survival was five months. Since the introduction of cyclophosphamide combined with corticosteroids, remission rates are in excess of 90%. Plasma exchange has proved beneficial for those patients with a rapidly progressive glomerulonephritis or lung haemorrhage.

The differential diagnosis of a collapsed nasal bridge with intact overlying skin includes:
1. Wegener's granulomatosis
2. Relapsing polychondritis
3. Congenital syphilis
4. Lepromatous leprosy.

a) What is the abnormal sign?
b) What is the likely underlying diagnosis in this 60-year-old man?

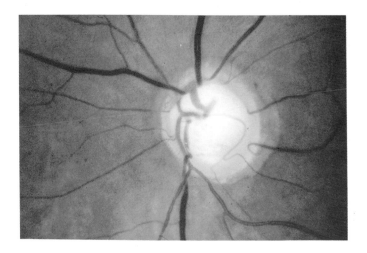

Answer to question 32

a) Cupping of the optic disc. The cup is enlarged and the vessels dip over the edge.

b) Chronic simple glaucoma, a common cause of blindness in the elderly. The disease is due to an increase in the resistance of outflow of aqueous humour within the trabecular meshwork. Chronic simple glaucoma is characterized by raised intraocular pressure (20–30 mmHg), increased cupping of the optic discs (often the earliest sign), and insidious painless loss of vision. An arcuate scotoma is the classical early visual field defect noted.

This is the peripheral blood film from an asymptomatic 35-year-old man in whom a raised white cell count was found during a routine medical check-up. Examination of his abdomen revealed 6 cm splenomegaly.

a) What abnormalities are present on the blood film and what is the likely diagnosis?

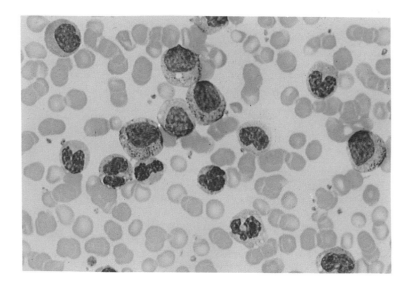

a) The blood film shows an increased number of neutrophils, one myelocyte and a basophil. The diagnosis is chronic myeloid leukaemia (CML) and this may be confirmed by demonstrating the presence of the Philadelphia chromosome in blood or bone marrow. An increased neutrophil count coupled with the presence of immature myeloid precursors and basophilia in the peripheral blood is a typical presentation of CML. Basophilia is a feature of myeloproliferative disorders in general and may be striking in CML.

Leukaemoid reactions, in which there is a marked leukocytosis (usually greater than $50\,000 \times 10^9$ l) and immature myeloid precursors circulate in the peripheral blood, can be seen associated with sepsis, carcinoma of the lung or stomach, Hodgkin's disease or dermatitis herpetiformis. Very occasionally the blood film may be difficult to differentiate from that seen in CML. However in a leukaemoid reaction the neutrophils usually show toxic granulation and Dohle bodies which are absent in CML, and the karyotype in a leukaemoid reaction is normal. Other useful laboratory indicators in favour of a diagnosis of CML are a low neutrophil alkaline phosphatase, a raised serum urate and an elevated level of vitamin B$_{12}$ and its binding protein transcobalamin.

The Philadelphia chromosome is formed by a reciprocal translocation of the distal part of the long arms of chromosome 9 and 22. This causes the abl gene, normally present on chromosome 9, to move to a position adjacent to the bcr gene on chromosome 22 resulting in the formation of a novel bcrabl gene. This new gene codes for a 210 kD protein with tyrosine kinase activity which is likely to be involved in the pathogenesis of CML. A Philadelphia chromosome is occasionally found in acute lymphoblastic leukaemia where it codes for a similar but smaller protein.

This 60-year-old woman presented with fever and splinter
haemorrhages.
a) What is the diagnosis?
b) How would you manage the patient?

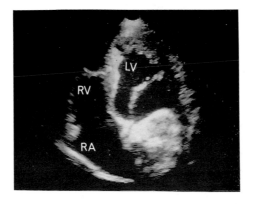

a) Left atrial myxoma. This is an apical four-chamber view of the heart which shows a large echogenic mass filling the left atrium. LV = Left ventricle, M = Myxoma, RA = Right atrium, RV = Right ventricle

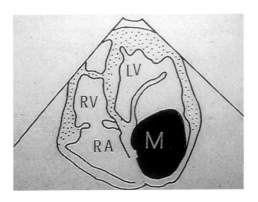

Although atrial myxomas are rare, they are the commonest primary cardiac neoplasm. These tumours are usually benign and recurrence after surgery reflects inadequate removal; occasionally cardiac myxomas are multiple. They are more common in females than in males. Three quarters arise from the fossa ovalis and are in the left atrium; the rest occur in the right atrium apart from very rare ventricular lesions. Macroscopically, myxomas are pedunculated and covered in adherent thrombus.

They may mimic other systemic diseases. Important clinical presentations include:

1. The symptoms and signs of left atrial outflow obstruction, i.e. a differential diagnosis of mitral stenosis
2. Systemic embolization, often when the patient is in sinus rhythm
3. As a pyrexia of unknown origin.

Cardiovascular signs are usually non-specific. Classically, signs including mitral systolic and diastolic murmurs change with posture. Rarely a tumour 'plop' may be heard in early diastole. Finger clubbing may complicate chronic cases.

Haematological findings include an elevated ESR, a normochromic normocytic anaemia, leukocytosis and thrombocytosis. There may be evidence of haemolysis.

b) Echocardiography is the investigation of choice. Once the diagnosis is confirmed urgent full thickness surgical excision is indicated. Regular echocardiographic follow-up is indicated as the rate of recurrence is up to 5% of cases.

This man presented to the accident and emergency department with abdominal pain.
a) What sign is shown and what is the diagnosis?
b) Give a differential diagnosis.
c) How would you confirm the diagnosis?

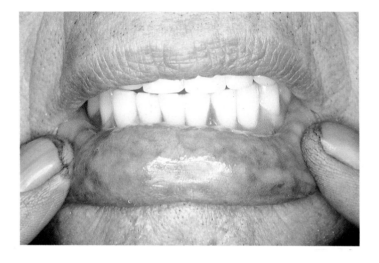

a) The slide shows the typical mucosal hyperpigmentation of Addison's disease (primary adrenal failure associated with increased levels of ACTH and β-MSH). Pigmentation is also seen

1. In the palmar creases
2. In areas of skin exposed to light or pressure, e.g. underneath bra straps
3. In scars acquired after the onset of Addison's disease.

Abdominal pain is a typical presenting feature of Addison's disease. Other clinical features include: weight loss, vomiting, diarrhoea, malaise, fever, vitiligo and muscle cramps. In females, loss of body hair occurs in both Addison's disease (due to loss of adrenal androgens) and secondary hypoadrenalism. In males, testicular androgens maintain body hair in Addison's disease.

A classic Addisonian crisis is characterized by hypotension, hyponatraemia, hyperkalaemia, an elevated urea and a metabolic acidosis. Hypoglycaemia may also be present though it is commoner with secondary hypoadrenalism caused by panhypopituitarism. Biochemistry may, however, be normal.

b) The differential diagnosis of Addison's disease includes:

1. Autoimmune Addison's disease
2. Tuberculous destruction of the adrenal glands
3. Granulomas
4. Metastatic carcinoma
5. Amyloidosis
6. Infarction of the adrenal cortex.

c) The diagnosis of Addison's disease is confirmed by demonstrating a low plasma cortisol which shows no diurnal variation and a raised plasma ACTH. Alternatively a synacthen test (tetracosactrin) may be performed. 1 mg of synacthen is given intramuscularly and blood drawn for plasma cortisol estimation at 4 and 24 hours.

SYNACTHEN TEST RESULTS:

- Normal — peak plasma cortisol > 1000 nmol/l at four hours
- Secondary hypoadrenalism — plasma cortisol levels greater at 24 than four hours
- Addison's disease — no response.

Adrenal autoantibodies may be detected in autoimmune Addison's disease.

Tuberculous destruction of the adrenal gland is often accompanied by adrenal calcification which is visible on a plain abdominal X-ray.

This 55-year-old woman complained of bilateral loss of vision.
a) What is the clinical sign shown here?
b) What is the diagnosis?

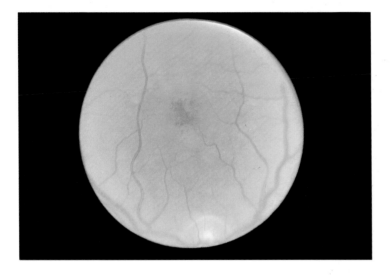

a) Diffuse macular pigmentation.
b) This patient has senile macular degeneration with pigmentation. Other causes include drugs such as chloroquine, and infections of the retina such as toxoplasma. Some patients with inherited adult onset cerebellar ataxia or other rare neurological diseases demonstrate macular pigmentation as a feature.

This is the peripheral blood film of a 35-year-old West African man who presented to casualty with excruciating bone pain.
a) What is the haematological abnormality?
b) What is the likely diagnosis?

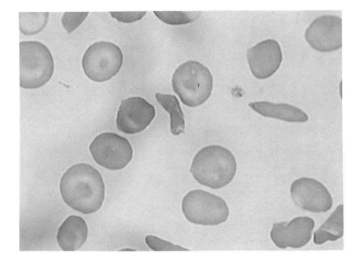

a) The blood film shows large numbers of target cells, characterized by their dense central staining, and the occasional irreversibly sickled cell.

b) The diagnosis is Hb SC disease. The diagnosis may be confirmed by haemoglobin electrophoresis which shows haemoglobins S and C present in approximately equal proportions.

Hb SC disease occurs in patients of West African descent. It usually runs a more benign course than homozygous sickle cell disease and may not be diagnosed until adulthood. In most cases there is a modest anaemia with mild splenomegaly and striking numbers of target cells seen on the blood film. The high haematocrit predisposes these patients to thrombotic complications, principally aseptic necrosis of the femoral and humeral heads and a proliferative retinopathy.

Causes of target cells include:

1. Haemoglobinopathies: Hb SS, thalassaemia
2. Iron deficiency
3. Hyposplenism
4. Obstructive liver disease.

a) This organism was isolated from a child who presented with abdominal pain and vomiting. What is the diagnosis?
b) What are the other recognized clinical features and complications?
c) How would you manage this case?

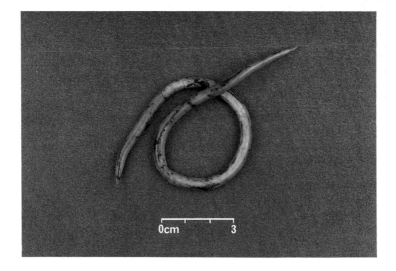

a) The worm is *Ascaris lumbricoides*, a recognized cause of intestinal obstruction particularly in children.

The gravid female worm, which may be 35 cm in length, lives in the human small intestine and can produce 200 000 eggs a day. Following ingestion, larvae hatch from the eggs, penetrate the wall of the small intestine and enter the circulation. After they reach the lungs, the larvae enter the alveoli, migrate up the bronchi and eventually reach the epiglottis. They are then swallowed and develop into adult worms which fix in the intestine to complete the cycle. In untreated cases, the adult worm survives one year and is then spontaneously expelled from the gut.

b) *A. lumbricoides* infection may be asymptomatic. Infected children who have high worm loads generally exhibit signs of malnutrition, general malaise and have occasional fevers. Recognized complications include:

1. Löeffler's syndrome: eosinophilic pneumonitis and bronchospasm caused by larval migration through the lungs; chest radiography shows diffuse shadowing and a peripheral blood film shows marked eosinophilia. Symptoms settle after 7–10 days unless reinfection occurs.
2. Intestinal obstruction as in this case
3. Ectopic migration of worms through the biliary tract may result in biliary obstruction and secondary cholangitis.

c) The diagnosis is made clinically and usually confirmed by detecting eggs in the faeces; occasionally an adult worm is seen in the stools. Barium examinations may outline the adult worms in the intestine.

Effective drugs include pyrantel pamoate, mebendazole, levamisole and piperazine salts. Many cases of intestinal obstruction will respond to conservative treatment and chemotherapy, though surgical intervention may be necessary.

Question 39

This 40-year-old man presents with these painful lumps.

a) What is the diagnosis?

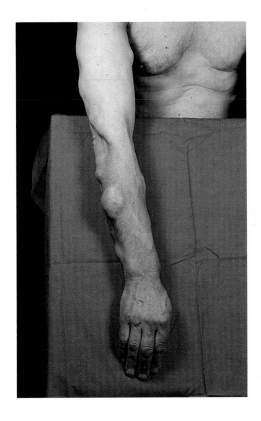

a) This patient has Dercum's disease, which is characterized by multiple painful lipomas. These may become massive and produce local complications. Malignant transformation is exceedingly rare. Surgical removal of the largest masses is the only treatment.

Lipomas are often multilobulated, and may be firm, rubbery or soft. They are deeper than epidermal cysts, and are mobile. Lipomas are also found in patients with Gardner's syndrome (multiple pre-malignant colonic adenomas, dermoids, epidermal cysts, fibromas and lipomas), Cowden's syndrome (sigmoid hamartomas), and MEN 1 (multiple endocrine neoplasia Type 1).

a) What is the diagnosis?
b) What are the complications of this disease and which groups of patients are most susceptible?

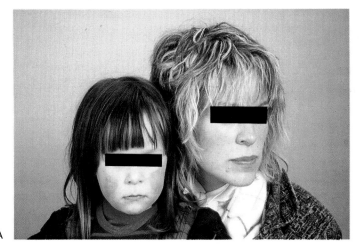

A

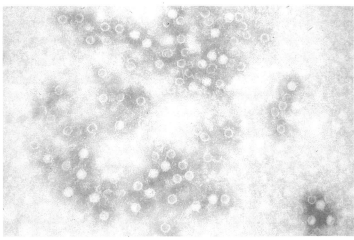

B

a) Erythema infectiosum caused by parvovirus B19. The electron micrograph shows small, round, 25 nm parvovirus particles. Parvovirus is a common infection in schoolchildren which usually presents as erythema infectiosum, the slapped cheek appearance shown in the slide, and a reticulate centripetal rash. Apart from rashes, children often have few other symptoms. Adult parvovirus infection however may be accompanied by flu-like symptoms, conjunctivitis, lymphadenopathy, splenomegaly, a self-limiting acute polyarthropathy and the rash described.

Acute parvovirus infection is confirmed by serology, and as in this case, viral particles may be identified in early serum samples.

b) Parvovirus infects and may lyse red cell progenitors. Patients with chronic haemolytic anaemias such as sickle cell anaemia or hereditary spherocytosis who contract parvovirus may develop aplastic crisis. Recovery of the bone marrow usually occurs after 5–10 days, accompanied by a reticulocytosis and a leukocytosis.

Parvovirus infection in immunocompromised patients may be associated with a chronic anaemia.

Transplacental transmission occurs and may rarely result in fetal death.

This 50-year-old man complains of marked pruritus. What is the diagnosis?

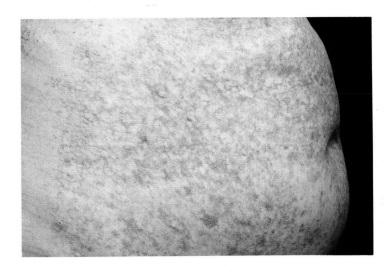

Mycosis fungoides. The slide shows the appearance of poikiloderma atrophicans vasculare.

Mycosis fungoides is a cutaneous T-cell lymphoma, which typically presents in the fourth or fifth decade. Skin biopsies reveal mycosis fungoides cells (Sézary cells), T lymphocytes and other inflammatory cells in the dermis. As the disease advances these cells are also seen in the epidermis where they constitute the microabscesses of Pautrier.

Mycosis fungoides may be classified by stage. Poikiloderma atrophicans vasculare is the early pre-malignant stage characterized by erythema, reticulate pigmentation, telangiectasia and atrophy. Some early lesions resemble a non-specific eczematous rash. The disease may progress slowly, over 10–20 years, to an infiltrative malignant stage with multiple indurated plaques. Eventually large bluish nodules develop, which may ulcerate and discharge. Finally dissemination occurs; large numbers of mycosis fungoides cells appear in the blood and there may be lymphadenopathy and hepatosplenomegaly.

Topical steroids, topical nitrogen mustard and PUVA have been used to treat early pre-infiltrative stages; superficial X-ray therapy and chemotherapeutic agents such as methotrexate or cyclophosphamide have been used for later stages of the disease.

This 25-year-old farmer's wife presented with a 2 week history of painful finger.
a) What is the diagnosis?
b) What other conditions can give this appearance?
c) What is your management?

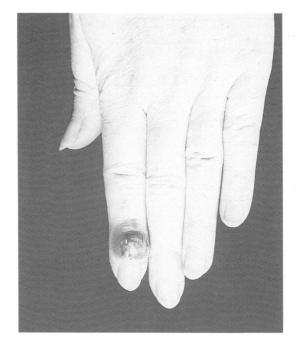

a) This patient has orf virus infection. This virus is one of the pox viruses.

b) Paronychial infections with candida, streptococcus and staphylococcus may look similar to this.

c) Patients with orf should be reassured, spontaneous resolution usually occurs.

The pox viruses are large DNA viruses. Variola (smallpox) was eradicated by vaccination programmes in 1980, and supplies of this virus are only kept in military laboratories. Vaccination with the cowpox virus (vaccinia) is not routine.

This is the peripheral blood film and Perls' stain of bone marrow
from a 50-year-old man with anaemia.
a) What abnormalities are present and what is the diagnosis?

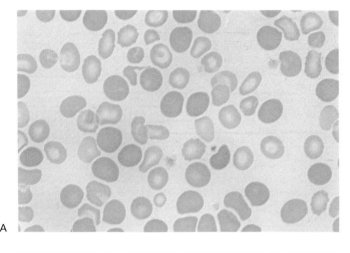

A

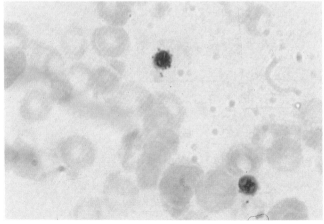

B

a) The blood film is dimorphic and the bone marrow shows ring sideroblasts. The diagnosis is sideroblastic anaemia. Differential diagnosis of a dimorphic blood film includes:

1. Sideroblastic anaemia
2. Recent blood transfusion
3. Treated iron deficiency
4. Mixed iron and folate or B_{12} deficiency.

Sideroblastic anaemias are a group of disorders characterized by increased numbers of ring sideroblasts in the bone marrow. Ring sideroblasts owe their appearance to the abnormal deposits of iron in perinuclear mitochondria which form a blue-green collar around the nucleus when stained with Perls' stain. The peripheral blood film in sideroblastic anaemia is dimorphic with a population of hypochromic microcytic cells caused by the underlying abnormality in haem synthesis. Despite the presence of this population the anaemia is commonly macrocytic.

Congenital (usually X-linked) sideroblastic anaemia is rare but may respond well to pyridoxine. There is a wide range of causes of acquired sideroblastic anaemia. Drugs, particularly alcohol, are an important and potentially reversible cause. Most cases of acquired sideroblastic anaemia however are idiopathic and classified with the myelodysplastic syndrome.

CLASSIFICATION OF SIDEROBLASTIC ANAEMIAS

1. Congenital
   — X-linked (rare)
2. Acquired
   — Idiopathic (myelodysplastic syndrome)
   — Alcohol
   — Drug induced, e.g. isoniazid, chloramphenicol
   — Lead
   — Rheumatoid arthritis
   — Myeloma.

Drugs are an important cause of sideroblastic anaemia. Most cases of acquired sideroblastic anaemia are idiopathic and are classified within the myelodysplastic syndromes. They usually present as a macrocytic anaemia with additional neutropenia or thrombocytopenia. If there is no response to a trial of pyridoxine, and drug-induced sideroblastic anaemia has been excluded, treatment usually consists of blood transfusion with iron chelation where appropriate.

On routine examination by his company doctor this man was found to have a diastolic murmur and was referred to outpatients.
a) What physical signs are shown in slides A and B?
b) What is the likely cause of the diastolic murmur and what is the diagnosis?
c) What other complications may occur?

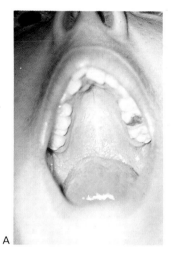

A

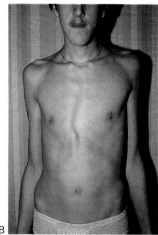

B

a) Slide A — a high arched palate.
Slide B — depressed twisted sternum.
b) Aortic incompetence. The combination of a high arched palate and aortic valve disease suggests a diagnosis of Marfan's syndrome.
c) Marfan's syndrome is inherited as an autosomal dominant trait with variable penetrance. Clinical features include: long thin extremities with span greater than height; arachnodactyly; depressed, twisted sternum; high arched palate; scoliosis; upward dislocation of the lens; joint and ligamentous laxity; herniae; aortic valve incompetence; aortic dissection; and mitral valve prolapse. Aortic root and valve disease is the main cause of death, though aortic surgery is often successfully performed in these patients.

NB: Homocystinuria, an autosomal recessive inborn error of metabolism, is phenotypically similar to Marfan's syndrome. Clinical features of homocystinuria include: Marfanoid body habitus; downward dislocation of the lens; low IQ; osteoporosis; vascular thrombosis; and livedo reticularis. Cardiac complications do not occur in homocystinuria.

This patient has a normal T4 and TSH.
a) What is the diagnosis?
b) How would you confirm the diagnosis?
c) What complications may arise?
d) What are the treatment options?

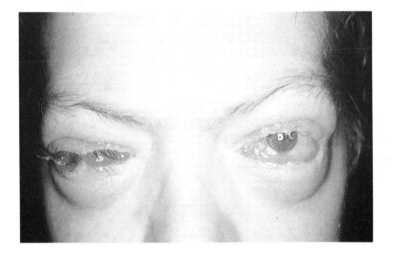

a) Acute malignant ophthalmic Graves' disease. Features on this slide are: proptosis and marked bilateral chemosis and oedema of the lids. 'Malignant' refers to the serious risk of loss of sight. Lid lag, lid retraction and external ophthalmoplegia are the other common signs of thyroid eye disease.
Ophthalmic Graves' disease may occur in hypothyroid, euthyroid or hyperthyroid patients. Overall, 70% of patients have some evidence of thyroid gland dysfunction. The condition is usually bilateral but may be asymmetrical or unilateral. Histology shows infiltration of the external ocular muscles with lymphocytes and oedema. Circulating antibodies to ocular muscle, found in many patients, have a disputed role in pathogenesis.
b) The swollen muscles may be visualized by CT scan allowing a firm diagnosis to be made.
The differential diagnosis of asymmetrical or unilateral proptosis includes:

1. Ophthalmic Graves' disease
2. Neoplasia
3. Cavernous sinus thrombosis
4. Caratico-cavernous fistula
5. Orbital cellulitis.

NB: Proptosis which is asymmetrical by more than 5 mm suggests a cause other than Graves' ophthalmopathy.
c) Complications include: corneal ulceration; keratitis; optic nerve compression; and ophthalmoplegia with diplopia. Compression of the optic nerve is often associated with only mild proptosis and may present with loss of acuity, field defects, colour loss or papilloedema.
d) Treatment:

1. Measures to protect the cornea, e.g. methylcellulose eye drops, eye pads, lateral tarsorrhaphy
2. Control of hyperthyroidism when present
3. Treatment with high dose corticosteroids (dexamethesone 4 mg q.d.s.) if the ocular features are severe or progressive, followed by urgent orbital decompression if there is no response; orbital irradiation has also been used for progressive disease
4. Fresnel prisms are useful for symptomatic diplopia; persistent diplopia may eventually require surgery.

a) What investigation is shown here?
b) What causes this type of defect?

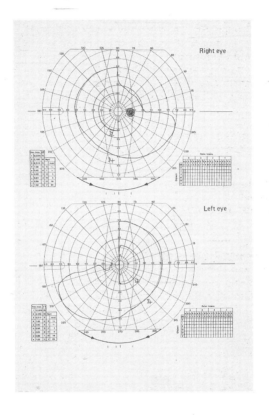

a) This is a Goldman perimetry, which documents visual field defects.

b) The defect shown here is upper quadrantic bitemporal hemianopia, which is found with chiasmal lesions. The most common causes are pituitary adenoma, craniopharyngioma or suprasellar meningioma. Other rare causes are optic glioma, cysts, vascular lesions, demyelinating diseases, trauma, Langerhans' cell granulomatosis (histiocytosis X), metastatic diseases, teratoma, arachnoiditis and cerebral infarction.

This 40-year-old woman presented with tinnitus and deafness.
a) What is the radiological abnormality?
b) What is the most likely diagnosis?

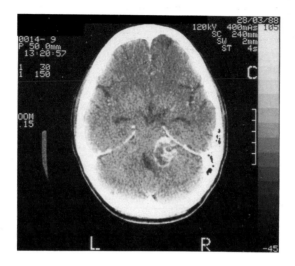

a) There is a well demarcated enhancing lesion in the region of the right cerebellopontine angle.
b) A right acoustic neuroma.

Acoustic neuromas are the commonest lesions occurring in the cerebellopontine angle. Other causes of cerebellopontine angle lesions include: meningioma; cholesteatoma; haemangioblastoma; neuromas affecting the fifth, seventh and tenth cranial nerves; aneurysm of the basilar artery; medulloblastoma; lymphomatous deposits; and nasopharyngeal carcinoma.

The cerebellopontine angle (triangle) comprises the cerebellum, lateral pons and inner third of the petrous bone. Lesions affect the fifth, sixth, seventh, eighth and ninth cranial nerves.

Acoustic neuromas arise from the vestibular division of the eighth cranial nerve, and commonly present in the fourth and fifth decades. The tumours are usually well encapsulated and unilateral; bilateral lesions occur, particularly in association with Von Recklinghausen's disease.

The effects of pressure on the immediate structures around the neuroma predominate; raised intracranial pressure is a late feature. Tinnitus and deafness are the earliest symptoms, followed by vertigo. Loss of the corneal reflex, as the trigeminal nerve is lifted up by the neuroma, is usually the earliest sign detected, followed by numbness in the distribution of the fifth nerve. Other signs include decreased auditory acuity, canal paresis on vestibular testing, and later paresis of the sixth, seventh and ninth nerves (although the seventh nerve is remarkably resilient to compression). Late manifestations include ipsilateral cerebellar signs and brain stem compression.

This is the blood film of a 16-year-old who presented with sore throat, jaundice and splenomegaly.
a) What is the haematological abnormality and what is the most likely diagnosis?
b) How would you confirm the diagnosis?
c) List the other haematological manifestations of this disease.

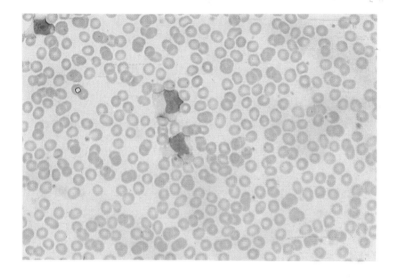

a) There are frequent atypical lymphocytes present on the blood film. The patient had infectious mononucleosis. Atypical lymphocytes are T cells reactive against B cells infected with the Epstein–Barr virus (EBV) and are morphologically characterized by their large amounts of pale blue cytoplasm which appears to flow around any surrounding erythrocytes. The greatest numbers of atypical lymphocytes are seen between the seventh and tenth days of the illness. Atypical lymphocytes are also seen with cytomegalovirus, influenza, toxoplasmosis and viral hepatitis A.

b)

1. The detection of high titre heterophil antibodies against sheep red blood cells (Paul–Bunnell test). Peak titres are reached during the second and third weeks and remain elevated for six weeks. Such antibodies may also be found in normal controls and in patients with serum sickness. Differential absorption studies distinguish the antibodies present in infectious mononucleosis, which are absorbed out by ox red blood cells but not guinea pig kidney; in contrast the antibodies in normal and serum sickness patients are absorbed by guinea pig kidney and not ox red cells.
2. A definitive diagnosis may be made by demonstrating a rise in titre of IgM antiviral capsid antibody.

c) Other haematological manifestations of EBV infection include:

1. Haemolytic anaemia: haemolysis occurs in 5% of patients but is usually mild and compensated. The antibody causing haemolysis is usually a cold reacting anti-i.
2. Thrombocytopenia: mild thrombocytopenia is common but a picture similar to idiopathic thrombocytopenic purpura lasting weeks and associated with an antiplatelet antibody is also seen.
3. Agranulocytosis is a very rare complication.

Note: Clinical features of infectious mononucleosis include: fever; malaise; headaches; neck stiffness; photophobia; morbilliform rash; bilateral cervical lymphadenopathy (75%); generalized lymphadenopathy (50%); splenomegaly (50%); hepatic involvement (abnormal liver function tests are common, clinical jaundice — 5%); and hepatomegaly (15%). In nearly all patients administration of ampicillin/amoxycillin is associated with the appearance of an itchy maculopapular rash.

Describe the abnormalities present in:
a) Slide A
b) Slide B
c) Slide C

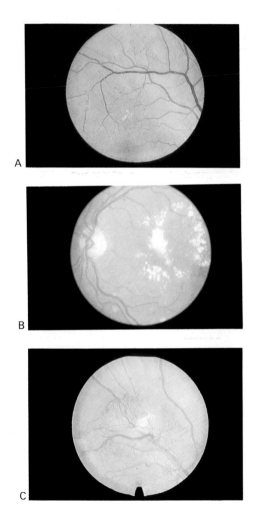

a) Background diabetic retinopathy with microaneurysms, haemorrhages and hard exudates.
b) Maculopathy — ring of hard exudates around the macula.
c) Proliferative retinopathy — a leash of new vessels is clearly visible.

Diabetic eye disease is the commonest cause of blindness in the United Kingdom between the ages of 20 and 65 years. Diabetic retinopathy is present in approximately 25% of cases of juvenile onset insulin-dependent diabetes after 10 years and approximately 50% of adult non-insulin-dependent diabetic patients after 10 years.

CLASSIFICATION OF DIABETIC EYE DISEASE:

1. Background retinopathy
   — Visual acuity is unaffected
   — Microaneurysms (outpouchings of retinal capillary wall)
   — Dot and blot haemorrhages
   — Retinal oedema
   — Hard exudates (represent leakage of lipid and lipoproteins)
2. Diabetic maculopathy (commoner in non-insulin-dependent diabetics)
   — Oedema, exudates and ischaemia affecting the macula
   — Central vision is lost, peripheral vision is maintained
3. Preproliferative retinopathy
   — Cotton wool spots (hold up of axonoplasmic flow, evidence of microvascular ischaemia)
4. Proliferative retinopathy
   — Neovascularization (develops in response to ischaemia)
   — The new vessels are liable to haemorrhage into the vitreous with subsequent fibrosis, retinal detachment and loss of vision
5. Rubeosis iridis
   — New vessel formation on the surface of the iris, may be complicated by glaucoma
6. Cataracts
   — Senile cataracts
   — Snow flake cataract of poorly controlled juvenile diabetes.

TREATMENT OF DIABETIC EYE DISEASE

Maculopathy due to hard exudate deposits can be successfully treated if caught early by focal photocoagulation of the leaking vessels adjacent to the macula.

Neovascularization of the retina as seen in slide C is an indication for argon laser panretinal photocoagulation.

a) What is the radiological abnormality and what is the most likely diagnosis?
b) List three other chronic complications of this disease.
c) How would you determine if there was active disease?

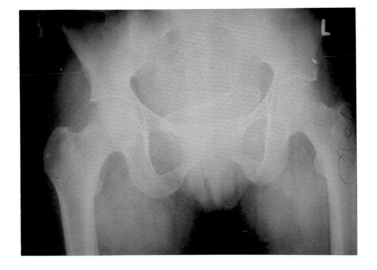

a) Calcification within the bladder wall caused by chronic infection
with *Schistosoma haematobium*.
Schistosomiasis is caused by trematodes. There are three
common species:

1. *S. haematobium* (Africa and the Middle East)
2. *S. mansoni* (Africa, South America and the Caribbean)
3. *S. japonicum* (Orient and South East Asia).

The fresh water larvae (cercariae) penetrate the skin and migrate to
the lungs and then the liver where they mature. The adult worms
migrate to their final habitat: in the case of *S. mansoni* and *S.
japonicum* the venules of the intestines and in the case of *S.
haematobium* the venules of the ureter and bladder. Eggs produced
reach fresh water via the urine or faeces and hatch into ciliated
miracidia which infect particular species of snails (intermediate
hosts) to complete the cycle.
   Penetration of the skin by cercariae may cause a hypersensitivity
rash (swimmer's itch). Three to eight weeks after infection, acute
schistosomiasis develops with headache, fever, myalgia,
hepatosplenomegaly, lymphadenopathy, urticaria and eosinophilia.
Symptoms of acute schistosomiasis are common with *S. japonicum*,
rare with *S. mansoni* and extremely rare with *S. haematobium*.

b) Complications of chronic schistosomiasis depend on the species:

1. Urinary (*S. haematobium*): ureteric and bladder fibrosis; bladder
   wall calcification; carcinoma of the bladder; hydronephrosis;
   renal failure; haemospermia in men and sterility in women
2. Liver (*S. mansoni, S. japonicum*): intrahepatic portal
   hypertension; hepatosplenomegaly; and the development of
   portal–systemic collaterals. Liver function tests are usually
   normal. It is debatable whether schistosomiasis alone causes
   cirrhosis or liver failure
3. Lung (severe disease is a feature of *S. mansoni* and *S.
   japonicum*): pulmonary hypertension and cor pulmonale
4. Central nervous system: *S. japonicum* typically affects the brain
   and is a common cause of focal epilepsy; it is rarely responsible
   for a generalized encephalitic illness. *S. mansoni* and *S.
   japonicum* may affect the spinal cord causing a transverse
   myelitis
5. Systemic amyloidosis.

c) Definitive diagnosis is made by finding viable eggs in the urine or
faeces, or by biopsying the bladder wall or rectum. The eggs of
each species are distinctive: *S. mansoni* — ellipsoidal eggs with a
lateral spine; *S. haematobium* — ellipsoidal eggs with a terminal
spine; and *S. japonicum* — spheroidal eggs with a small knob.

Praziquantel is the drug of choice; following treatment many chronic
and apparently irreversible lesions will improve.

This 30-year-old lady developed a rash in the second trimester of her third pregnancy. What is the diagnosis?

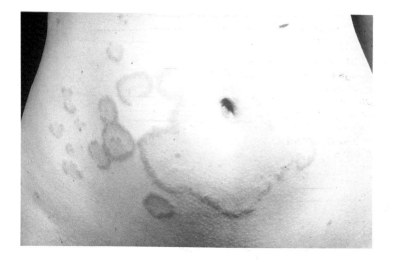

Herpes gestationis is a rare, pruritic, bullous disease of pregnancy. The rash may occur during the first pregnancy but usually is seen in the second or third trimester of subsequent pregnancies. Bullous lesions develop on the hands and around the umbilicus and the mouth. Lesions usually resolve two to three weeks after delivery. The disease tends to recur with increasing severity in successive pregnancies. Exacerbations may occur premenstrually or with the oral contraceptive pill.

Treatment is with systemic corticosteroids. Histology shows that blisters form above the basement membrane; direct immunofluorescence reveals C3 and IgG deposition along the basement membrane. Placental transfer of IgG antibodies can cause a self-limiting bullous rash in the neonate.

This person presented with grand mal convulsions.
a) What is the diagnosis?
b) How would you confirm the diagnosis?

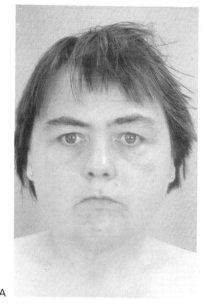

A

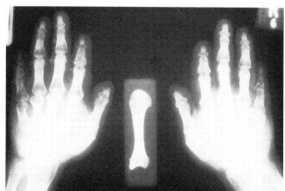

B

a) Pseudohypoparathyroidism — an inherited end organ resistance to PTH. The mode of inheritance is variable; some families show an X-linked dominant pattern. Features include short stature, a round face, short metacarpals and metatarsal bones (typically the fourth and fifth digits). Patients are often of low intelligence. Associated disorders include hypothyroidism, diabetes mellitus and gonadal dysgenesis.

Serum biochemistry shows hypocalcaemia, hyperphosphataemia, an elevated PTH level and normal serum creatinine and vitamin D levels.

Symptoms and signs of hypocalcaemia include: paraesthesiae; carpopedal spasm; abdominal cramps; irritability; papilloedema; and ectopic calcification (basal ganglia are a favoured site).

Slide A shows the typical facial appearance and slide B the short metacarpal bones. The convulsions are likely to be due to hypocalcaemia.

b) The diagnosis may be confirmed by dynamic endocrine testing. A PTH infusion normally results in an increase in plasma and urine cAMP along with phosphaturia. Two types of pseudohypoparathyroidism can be identified using this test, which reflect complete or partial end organ resistance to PTH: Type 1 no change in phosphate excretion, urine cAMP levels do not rise; Type 2 no change in phosphate excretion, urine cAMP levels rise.

This 25-year-old soldier presented with fever and arthralgia, and a diastolic murmur.
a) What clinical sign is shown?
b) What is the underlying diagnosis?
c) How would you manage this patient?

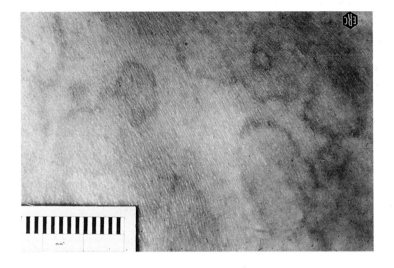

a) The typical appearance of erythema marginatum is shown.

b) This patient has two major criteria (Ducket Jones criteria) for the diagnosis of rheumatic fever. The other major criteria are: polyarthritis, usually affecting large joints of the legs, particularly the knees; subcutaneous nodules; and chorea. Minor criteria are fever, arthralgia, previous rheumatic fever, raised ESR, CRP or extended PR interval. Two major or one major and two minor criteria are sufficient for the diagnosis, on condition that prior streptococcal infection can be demonstrated, either by showing a rise in ASO titre, or by culture of group A streptococci.

c) High dose aspirin is used during acute infection. Steroids are also used in certain cases, starting at 40–60 mg of prednisolone. The most important point is prevention of subsequent infection with rheumatogenic strains of streptococci. Traditionally, this disease is found in children between the ages of 5 and 15, and a monthly injection of 1.2 million units of benzathine penicillin G is effective prophylaxis. Oral sulphonamides or penicillins are less effective, and erythromycin is used in allergic patients. Prophylaxis is given until the age of 20, or for at least 5 years. Since this disease is seen much later in developed countries recommendations are less clear. Reinfection should be prevented, since cardiac damage is usually caused by reinfection. In developed countries, patients often present with rheumatic valve lesions without a prior history of rheumatic fever.

This 60-year-old man presented with weight loss and diarrhoea.
a) What clinical sign is demonstrated here?
b) How would you manage the patient?

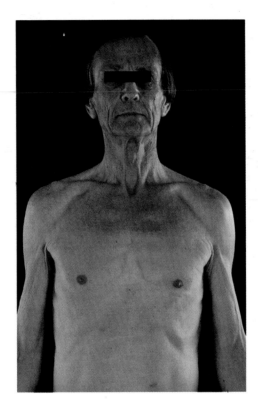

a) A carcinoid flush is shown here. The flush can result in chronic facial oedema and telangiectasia in some patients. Food, alcohol, calcium, and pentagastrin can precipitate this reaction. Although several chemical substances such as histamine, serotonin, kallikreins, kinins and prostaglandins have been blamed for this reaction, it is unclear which of these is more important.

b) Management of carcinoid syndrome depends on whether the disease is localized or disseminated. Carcinoid flush is usually associated with metastatic disease, so this patient probably has disseminated disease. Some patients with malignant carcinoid have demonstrated deficiency of niacin, and even pellagra. This occurs because tryptophan is converted to 5-hydroxytamine, which is used to synthesize serotonin. Pyridoxine should be given, since it catalyses the conversion of tryptophan to niacin. In the event of a single localized mass, excision may be possible. Most carcinoid tumours are benign, since they are discovered in approximately 0.75% of autopsy series. Many carcinoids are however indolent, and the 5 year survival of patients with localized metastatic disease is 50%, while 30% of those with liver metastases survive 5 years or longer. Up to 10% of patients with liver metastases may live for 10 years or longer. Pharmacological therapy is useful: antihistamines, steroids, NSAIDs, and serotonin antagonists have been used. Intravenous or subcutaneous somatostatin is effective, particularly in those with diarrhoea.

The diagnosis of carcinoid is made by demonstrating the excretion of 30 mg or more of 5-hydroxyindoleacetic acid (5-HIAA) in a 24 hour urine sample. Patients should not use certain drugs before the test (phenothiazines, methenamine mandelate) or foods containing serotonin such as bananas, avocados and walnuts. Diseases such as bacterial overgrowth and coeliac disease may result in increased 5-HIAA levels.

Question 55

a) What are the abnormalities present on this blood film?
b) How would you investigate further?

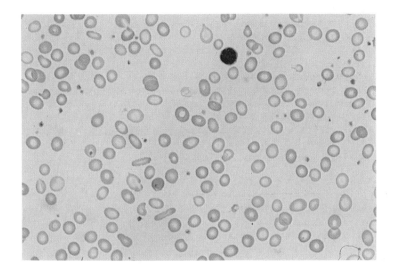

a) The red cells are hypochromic (they are extremely pale) and microcytic (the majority are considerably smaller than the normal lymphocyte).
Hypochromic anaemias are caused by abnormal synthesis of haemoglobin and this may be due to either iron deficiency, alpha or beta thalassaemia, or sideroblastic anaemia.

b) This blood film is from a patient with iron deficiency anaemia but it is not possible to differentiate between these diagnostic possibilities simply by looking at the blood film; a careful history (e.g. gastrointestinal symptoms, menorrhagia, ethnic origin, family and past medical history) and examination are essential. Investigation rests on assessment of iron status and haemoglobin electrophoresis if appropriate. Sideroblastic anaemia can only be diagnosed by a bone marrow aspirate with Perls' iron stain to look for ring sideroblasts.

This 60-year-old smoker complained of persistent cough and difficulty in climbing stairs.
a) Describe the rash.
b) What is the diagnosis?
c) What are the other recognized cutaneous manifestations?

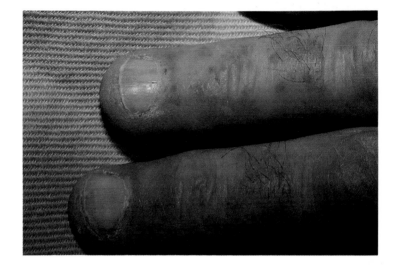

a) The purple plaques over the knuckles are Gottron's papules, a recognized cutaneous manifestation of dermatomyositis.
b) Dermatomyositis and carcinoma of the bronchus.
Dermatomyositis in patients over the age of fifty may be associated with underlying malignancy. The frequency of this association is subject to debate but the history of persistent cough in a smoker suggests the possibility of an underlying bronchial carcinoma.
c) Other cutaneous manifestations include:

1. Heliotropic rash on the eyelids, cheeks and light exposed areas
2. Nail fold changes with periungual erythema, cuticular hypertrophy and infarcts
3. Sclerodermatous skin changes with cutaneous and muscular calcification.

Diagnosis of dermatomyositis requires three out of the four diagnostic criteria for myositis to be present in addition to the typical dermatomyositis rash.
Criteria for the diagnosis of myositis are:

1. Proximal muscle weakness — usually symmetrical
2. Elevated serum levels of muscle enzymes
3. Typical muscle biopsy changes
4. The triad of electromyographic changes: polyphasic, short, small motor unit potentials; high frequency repetitive discharges; and spontaneous fibrillation.

Question 57

a) Name the physical signs present in slides A and B.
b) List the causes of each.

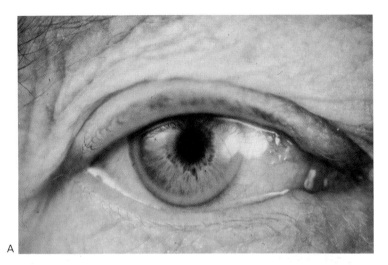

A

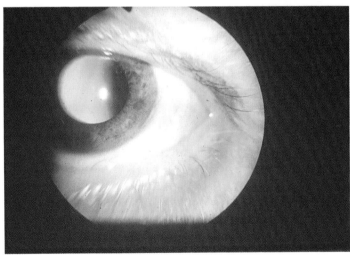

B

Answer to question 57

a) Slide A — corneal arcus. Corneal arcus is generally maximal at 6 and 12 o'clock.
Slide B — corneal calcification visible at 3 o'clock. Corneal calcification is maximal at 3 and 9 o'clock.
b) Corneal arcus differential diagnosis includes:

1. Old age
2. Hypercholesterolaemia (Type IIa, Type IIb).

Corneal calcification differential diagnosis includes:

1. Sarcoidosis
2. Hyperparathyroidism
3. Chronic renal failure
4. Vitamin D abuse.

Question 58

This 27-year-old man presented to his GP.
a) What is the clinical diagnosis?
b) Name some conditions associated with this.

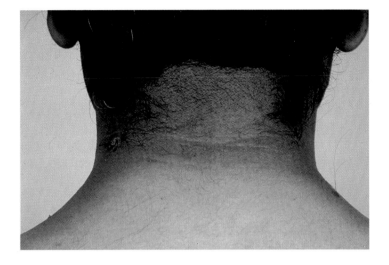

a) Acanthosis nigricans.
b) Recognized associations include:

1. Underlying malignancy: usually gastric adenocarcinoma, although squamous carcinoma can precede; acanthosis nigricans may be seen before or after the presentation with the malignancy
2. Obesity
3. Inherited
4. Endocrinological: diabetes mellitus, insulin resistance, lipodystrophy, Cushing's syndrome, acromegaly, polycystic ovary syndrome, hypothyroidism.

This 70-year-old man presented with progressive dysphagia.
a) What is the clinical sign shown?
b) Suggest a unifying diagnosis.

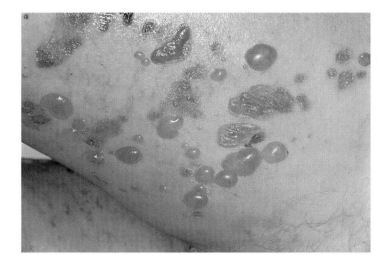

a) Large bullous lesions typical of the subepidermal blisters of pemphigoid are seen.

b) Pemphigoid may be associated with an underlying malignancy in 10% of patients. The progressive dysphagia in this patient suggests an oesophageal malignancy. Squamous carcinoma of the oesophagus was seen at oesophagoscopy.

Pemphigoid is less common but more benign than pemphigus vulgaris. Flexural areas are involved, and only rarely mucosa. Histology demonstrates C3 and immunoglobulin deposition at the dermo-epidermal junction. Antibodies to the hemidesmosome, which are usually IgG4, are found in 70% of patients. This antibody has been shown to recognize an antigen of between 180 and 230 kD. Steroid therapy (prednisone 0.5–1 mg/kg/day) is usually effective, and should be used for approximately 6 months.

   Pemphigus vulgaris often involves mucosa, and blisters are more superficial and fragile. High dose steroids (prednisone 1–2 mg/kg/day) result in mortality reduction. Azathioprine or cyclophosphamide may be used in conjunction with steroids. Mortality is approximately 5%.

a) What is the diagnosis?
b) How would you confirm the diagnosis?
c) How would you treat this 15-year-old boy?

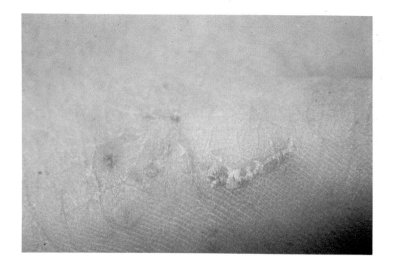

a) Scabies. The slide shows a typical burrow caused by the mite *Sarcoptes scabei*. Female mites, which can survive 36 hours away from the host, burrow into the epidermis and lay their eggs. Burrows are often sparse but may be seen in the web spaces of the fingers and the flexor aspects of the wrists. Burrows do not occur above the neck line, except in infants and immunosuppressed patients. Pruritus, worse at night, develops four to six weeks after infection when the patient develops a hypersensitivity reaction to the mite or its fomites leading to widespread excoriations. Urticarial papules generally only occur around the penis, buttocks, areolae and umbilicus.

b) The diagnosis is confirmed by identifying an adult female, obtained from an intradermal burrow with a needle. If burrows are difficult to find Cullen and Childers' test may be employed; topical tetracycline is taken up into burrows and will fluoresce yellow under Wood's light.

c) Treatment should be given to the index case and all close contacts. Agents used include lindane, malathiom and permethrin. Older agents, such as benzyl benzoate should be avoided in children.

Secondary bacterial infection, typically staphylococcus or streptococcus, is common, especially in the tropics; appropriate antibiotics should be given.

A highly contagious variant, Norwegian scabies, occurs in institutions and immunosuppressed patients and may lead to a hypertrophic psoriasiform rash.

This young man was admitted with fever and marked tachypnoea.
a) What is the diagnosis?
b) What conditions are associated with this diagnosis?

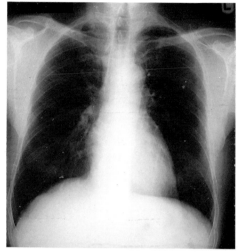

A

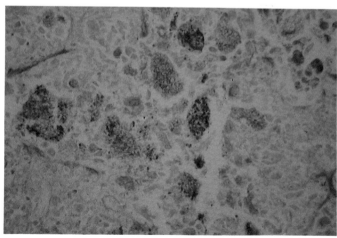

B

a) *Pneumocystis carinii* pneumonia.
Slide A — the chest X-ray is normal.
Slide B — the lung biopsy shows the presence of *Pneumocystis carinii* cysts.
b) Pneumocystis pneumonia occurs almost exclusively in immunocompromised patients. At least 60% of AIDS patients will eventually develop pneumocystis pneumonia.

Pneumocystis pneumonia typically presents with a gradual history of increasing shortness of breath, a non-productive cough, tachypnoea and low grade fever. At this early stage there are often no clinical signs and the chest X-ray is normal. Marked hypoxia is common and precedes radiological changes by several days. In advanced cases the chest X-ray shows diffuse bilateral alveolar shadowing.
The diagnosis is confirmed by finding the organisms in alveolar washings or, more dependably, in a lung biopsy. Pneumocystis stains poorly with conventional stains, therefore silver stains are essential to show the organisms clustered in the alveoli and being phagocytosed by macrophages.
Co-trimoxazole is the drug of choice, pentamidine isothionate is the alternative. Untreated cases of pneumocystis pneumonia have a fatality rate of approximately 100%; effective treatment reduces the fatality rate to 25%.
Antibodies are not useful in making the diagnosis since most normal people have antibodies by four years of age, following subclinical infection.

Question 62

This patient presented to her general practitioner complaining of persistent headaches.
a) What is the diagnosis? List the recognized clinical features.
b) How would you confirm the diagnosis?
c) What are the treatment options?

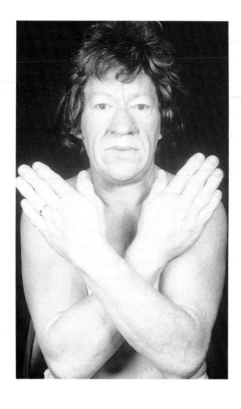

a) Acromegaly caused by excess growth hormone secreted by
pituitary adenoma.
Clinical features include: thickened greasy skin; enlargement of
skeleton with alteration in ring, hat and shoe size, etc.; prognathism;
hyperhidrosis; hirsutism; diabetes mellitus; hypertension;
cardiomyopathy; visceromegaly; entrapment neuropathy (e.g. carpal
tunnel syndrome); arthropathy; proximal myopathy; hypercalcuria;
hypercalcaemia; hyperphosphaturia. Local effects of tumour include:

1. Pressure on optic chiasm resulting in an upper quadrant
   bitemporal hemianopia
2. Pressure on the optic nerves
3. Lateral extension into cavernous sinus causing third, fourth of
   fifth cranial nerve palsies.

Headaches are common and are caused by local stretching of the
dura. Features related to high prolactin levels or hypopituitarism may
be present.

b) The diagnosis is confirmed by demonstrating elevated levels of
growth hormone (GH), which fails to suppress (< 4 mU/l) during
an oral glucose tolerance test. The prolactin levels are often
elevated. A lateral skull X-ray will show enlargement of the
pituitary fossa in 90% of cases. Computerized tomography can
identify a microadenoma and show the extent of tumour growth.
All patients should have their visual acuity tested and visual fields
accurately charted. Hypopituitarism should be excluded.

c) Treatment options are:

1. Bromocriptine, a dopamine antagonist, may be used to lower
   GH levels and improve symptoms prior to surgery.
   Bromocriptine may also be used as sole treatment in those in
   whom surgery is contraindicated. Somatostatin analogue given
   twice a day is also effective in lowering growth hormone levels.
2. Trans-sphenoidal hypophysectomy — for tumour confined to
   the fossa or with only small suprasellar extension. If growth
   hormone levels remain high post surgery, external radiotherapy
   may be given.
3. Transfrontal craniotomy, followed by external radiation, is
   undertaken for large suprasellar tumours.
4. External radiotherapy alone.
5. ^{90}Yttrium implants.

a) What is the diagnosis?
b) Give the differential diagnosis.
c) What visual symptoms may the patient complain of?

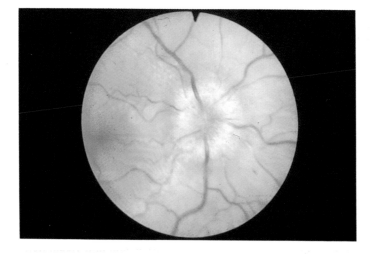

a) Papilloedema — the disc is pink and swollen with indistinct margins. In many cases the swollen disc is accompanied by venous engorgement and flame-shaped haemorrhages centred around the disc.

b) Causes of papilloedema include:

1. Raised intracranial pressure
2. Accelerated phase hypertension (Grade IV)
3. Retinal vein thrombosis
4. Carbon dioxide retention
5. Hypoparathyroidism
6. Exophthalmos
7. Vitamin A poisoning
8. Lead poisoning
9. Bacterial endocarditis.

c) Fleeting episodes of visual loss in one or both eyes, typically lasting a few seconds, are pathognomonic of papilloedema. Unlike acute papillitis, visual acuity is initially well maintained. Visual field changes accompanying papilloedema include enlargement of the blind spot and a concentric diminution in visual fields.

Papillitis — inflammation of the optic nerve head — is an important differential diagnosis. In papillitis, early loss of visual acuity is typical and accompanied by a large central scotoma.

a) What physical sign is demonstrated in slide A and what is the differential diagnosis?
b) What physical sign is shown in slide B?
c) What diagnosis encompasses signs A and B?

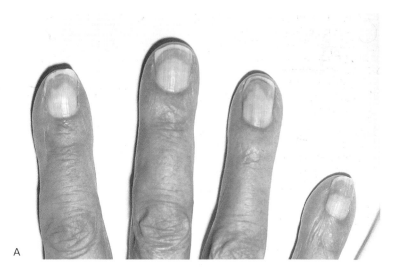

A

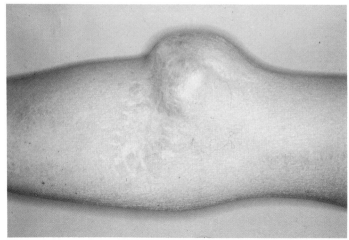

B

a) Leukonychia. The differential diagnosis of white nails includes:
1. Darier's disease
2. Renal failure
3. Hypoalbuminaemia: nephrotic syndrome; liver disease; protein-losing enteropathy
4. Arsenic/cytotoxic drugs
5. Fungal infection.

b) There is an arteriovenous forearm fistula with local aneurysm formation.

c) Dialysis-dependent chronic renal failure.

This man presented to his GP.
a) What is this sign?
b) What is the differential diagnosis?

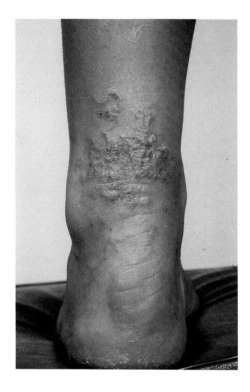

a) Larva migrans — the migration of larvae under the skin accompanied by urticarial wheals.

b) This syndrome results from worms or their larvae migrating through skin.

The differential diagnosis includes:

1. *Ancylostoma braziliense* and *A. caninum* (hookworms), intestinal parasites of dogs which cause larva migrans in man. The larvae progress irregularly at 1 cm/hour. The advancing end of the burrow is red and itchy, the older part brown and scaly. Treatment is by local application of thiabendazole.
2. *Strongyloides stercoralis* (a nematode) endemic in the tropics, especially the Far East. Man is the chief natural host. Clinical features include:
   — Local itch at the initial site of larval entry
   — Typical linear urticarial wheals (these may extend at the rate of 3 cm an hour and are hence referred to as 'larva currens'
   — Symptoms attributable to gut infestation, e.g. anaemia, diarrhoea, malabsorption, ileus and volvulus
   — Heavy infection which may be associated with asthma or alveolar haemorrhage. Strongyloides is best treated with oral thiabendazole or mebendazole.

Rare causes are:

1. *Gnathostoma*, a nematode found in South East Asia
2. *Paragonimus*, a lung fluke found in fresh water crustacea, especially in Asia
3. *Sparaganum*, a tapeworm larva found in South East Asia.

This 50-year-old man became acutely short of breath.
a) What is the diagnosis?
b) What clinical signs would you expect?
c) What treatment is indicated?

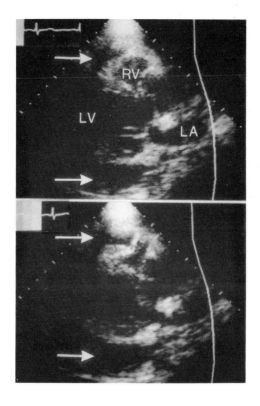

a) Pericardial effusion with cardiac tamponade. This slide shows parasternal long axis views from a patient with moderate pericardial effusion (arrows) during systole (top) and diastole (bottom). During diastole there is inward displacement of the right ventricular free wall.

b) Pericardial tamponade occurs when the pericardial pressure increases to a level which impedes ventricular filling. Clinical signs of tamponade include a sinus tachycardia, relative hypotension, peripheral vasoconstriction, a raised jugular venous pressure which increases further with inspiration (Kussmaul's sign), pulsus paradoxus in excess of 10 mmHg and quiet heart sounds.

c) Urgent pericardiocentesis should be undertaken using the subcostal or apical route. The electrocardiogram should be monitored throughout the procedure. For large effusions continuous drainage may be effected by inserting a temporary drain.

Question 67

This is the peripheral blood from a 46-year-old man who developed the itchy rash shown. His MCV is 109 fl.
a) What are the haematological abnormalities?
b) What is the rash and what is the likely aetiology?

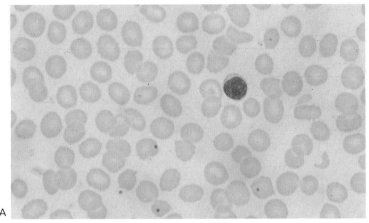

A

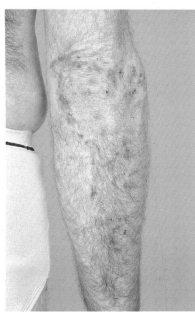

B

a) The peripheral blood shows Howell–Jolly bodies and oval
macrocytes.

b) Dermatitis herpetiformis, usually associated with gluten
sensitivity. The slide shows the typical itchy vesicobullous lesions
which are predominantly distributed over the extensor surfaces.
The rash is associated with granular deposition of IgA in the
dermis. The most likely diagnosis is coeliac disease.

Howell–Jolly bodies are a feature of any hyposplenic state and in
coeliac disease are caused by the associated splenic atrophy. Oval
macrocytes are typically present on the blood film and result from
folate deficiency due to the subtotal villous atrophy.

Coeliac disease is usually diagnosed in childhood but it may
present at any age, sometimes with minimal symptoms. Both folate
and iron deficiency are common and the MCV at presentation may
be normal, high or low. It is an important diagnosis to consider in
any adult with unexplained iron deficiency. The diagnosis is
suggested by villous atrophy seen on a duodenal or jejunal biopsy
and is confirmed if there is improvement on a gluten free diet.
Antiendomysial and antigliadin antibodies are a sensitive screening
test for the presence of coeliac disease provided the patient does not
have IgA deficiency.

Many patients with dermatitis herpetiformis respond to a gluten
free diet. Dapsone is effective in relieving itch, though side effects,
particularly haemolytic anaemia, limit its use.

a) What is the diagnosis?
b) How would you confirm the diagnosis?

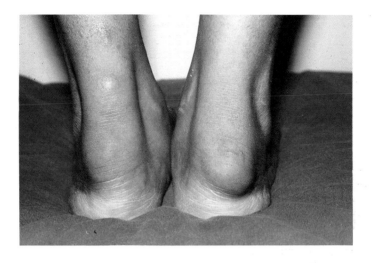

a) Tendon xanthomas over the Achilles tendon. Typically, tendon xanthomas occur in familial hypercholesterolaemia (WHO Type IIa). Tendon xanthomas are a very rare feature of secondary causes of hypercholesterolaemia.

Type IIa hypercholesterolaemia is characterized by raised low density lipoprotein levels (LDL), caused by a deficiency of LDL receptors on cell surfaces. Familial hypercholesterolaemia is inherited in an autosomal dominant fashion. Early onset ischaemic heart disease is the commonest mode of presentation and the average age span for untreated homozygotes is 20 years. Other clinical features include xanthelasma, corneal arcus and a polyarthritis.

b) Plasma lipid estimation will reveal hypercholesterolaemia reflecting increased LDL levels. The lipoprotein electrophoresis pattern is typically Type IIa; VLDL levels are usually normal or mildly elevated and HDL levels low.

a) What is the likely diagnosis in this 6-year-old boy?
b) How would you confirm your diagnosis?

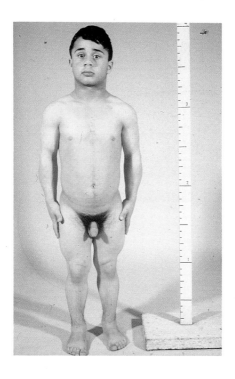

a) An 'Infant Hercules' — the most likely diagnosis is congenital adrenal hyperplasia. The slide shows a young boy with evidence of virilization but small testicles.

In constitutional precocious puberty (raised GnRH) or in patients with intracranial lesions (e.g. pinealoma, craniopharyngioma) which cause hypothalamic inhibition of the anterior pituitary to be lost, the genitals are adult-sized. An interstitial cell tumour of either testis might also present in this way, however the testis involved would be enlarged.

b) Congenital adrenal hyperplasia is an autosomal recessive inborn error of metabolism due to a deficiency or partial deficiency of one of the enzymes involved in the synthesis of cortisol.

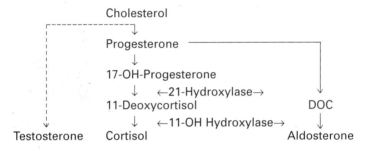

Cholesterol
↓
Progesterone
↓
17-OH-Progesterone
↓ ←21-Hydroxylase→
11-Deoxycortisol   DOC
↓ ←11-OH Hydroxylase→   ↓
Testosterone Cortisol   Aldosterone

The commonest enzymes involved are 21-hydroxylase or 11β-hydroxylase and, as shown, both are necessary for the synthesis of cortisol and aldosterone.

Partial deficiency of the 21-hydroxylase enzyme leads to low cortisol levels. A compensatory rise in ACTH tends to return cortisol levels to normal at the expense of stimulating the left hand pathway, resulting in androgen excess and virilization. Some infants with partial 21-hydroxylase deficiency will also be salt deficient; the severe cases present neonatally.

Deficiency of the 11-hydroxylase enzyme produces a similar picture of virilization but the subjects are hypertensive due to accumulation of 11-deoxycorticosterone (DOC).

Diagnosis depends on finding low or normal plasma cortisol, an inappropriately high plasma ACTH, raised androgens, and raised plasma and urinary 17-hydroxyprogesterone levels. Analysis of specific urinary metabolites defines the exact enzyme defect.

TREATMENT

Cortisol replacement, plus fludrocortisone if the patient is a salt loser. Failure to suppress androgen excess will lead to over-advancement of bone age with premature epiphyseal fusion and eventual stunting of growth.

This 30-year-old Turkish man presented with a right deep vein thrombosis.
a) What is the diagnosis?
b) What are the other recognized complications?

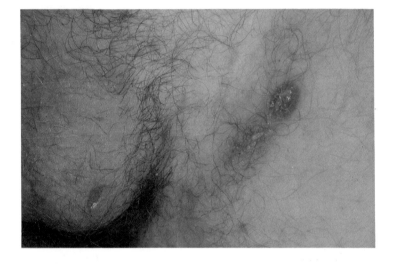

a) Behçet's syndrome. The combination of genital ulcers and deep vein thrombosis in a young Turkish man suggests Behçet's syndrome.

b) Behçet's syndrome is a rare multisystem vasculitic disorder which affects males more commonly than females. The syndrome is more common in patients from Turkey, Japan, Greece and the Middle East.

Clinical features include the triad first described by Behçet: recurrent oral aphthous ulceration; genital ulceration; and iritis.
Other clinical features include:

1. Fever and malaise
2. Eye lesions: episcleritis; papilloedema; optic atrophy
3. Skin lesions: cutaneous vasculitic lesions; erythema nodosum; the development of skin pustules at venepuncture sites (pathergy)
4. Polyarthritis
5. Vascular lesions: arterial and venous thrombosis; localized aneurysms
6. Gastrointestinal lesions: diarrhoea; abdominal pain; colonic ulcers
7. Central nervous system lesions: brain stem syndromes; organic confusional states; meningitis; myelitis
8. Pericarditis.

The diagnosis is a clinical one. Biopsies show a non-specific necrotizing small vessel vasculitis. The ESR is raised; a mild anaemia is common and circulating immune complexes may be detected.
In patients with Behçet's syndrome HLA B12 has been linked to recurrent oral ulcers and HLA B5 with ocular disease. Treatment is unsatisfactory, but corticosteroids and colchicine have been used with varying degrees of success.

Differential diagnosis of oral and genital ulcers:

1. Behçet's syndrome
2. Reiter's syndrome
3. Crohn's disease
4. Pemphigus vulgaris
5. Syphilis
6. Herpes simplex
7. Erythema multiforme
8. Strachan's syndrome (orogenital ulcers/sensory neuropathy/amblyopia — aetiology unknown).

This 40-year-old man presented with polydipsia and polyuria.
a) What is the clinical sign shown here?
b) What is the likely diagnosis, and how does this explain his presenting symptoms?

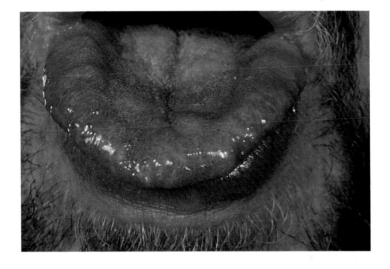

a) Multiple mucosal neuromas of the tongue and lips are seen.
b) This patient has MEN IIB (multiple endocrine neoplasia) syndrome. Some authorities call MEN IIB, MEN III syndrome. This syndrome is similar to MEN II (Sipple's syndrome), but differs in that mucosal neuromas of the lips, cheeks and tongue are characteristic. Gastrointestinal ganglioneuromas, neuromas, neurofibromas, and café au lait spots may be seen in MEN III. These patients may also have a Marfanoid appearance. Inheritance is autosomal dominant, but is often sporadic. C cell hyperplasia is found in 100% as in MEN II, and medullary thyroid cancer is seen in both. Parathyroid cell hyperplasia with hypercalcaemia is rare in MEN III, but is seen in approximately 20% of MEN II patients. This patient, however, did have hypercalcaemia as a result of parathyroid hyperplasia, resulting in hypercalcaemic renal damage, polyuria and polydipsia. The incidence of phaeochromocytoma is the same in MEN II and MEN III (20%).

MEN I (Werner's sydnrome) is characterized by parathyroid hyperplasia or adenomas (up to 95%), pancreatic adenoma in a third, and parathyroid adenoma in approximately 20%. Multiple lipomas are seen. Insulinomas are the most common pancreatic adenoma, but glucagonoma, gastrinoma (Zollinger–Ellison syndrome), somatostatinoma, and serotoninoma have been described. Inheritance is autosomal dominant.

This is the peripheral blood from an 86-year-old man with lymphadenopathy and a raised white cell count.
What is the likely diagnosis?

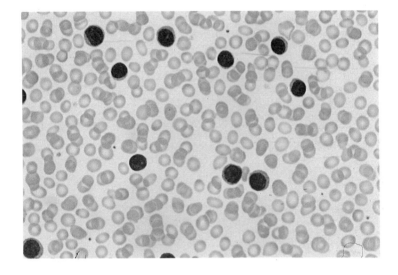

There is an increase in the number of morphologically normal lymphocytes; the diagnosis is chronic lymphatic leukaemia (CLL). This degree of lymphocytosis, in adults, is almost pathognomonic for CLL. A similar degree of lymphocytosis may be seen in children with pertussis.

Although the lymphocytes in CLL appear normal they are more fragile than normal and this results in the characteristic smear cells often seen on the blood film. The diagnosis can be confirmed by demonstrating a monoclonal population of lymphocytes in peripheral blood and marrow using cell surface markers.

Causes of a lymphocytosis include:

1. Infections:
   - Bacterial — pertussis
   - Viral — rubella, infectious mononucleosis, hepatitis
2. Chronic lymphatic leukaemia
3. Non-Hodgkin's lymphoma with peripheral blood overspill.

Haematological complications of chronic lymphatic leukaemia include:

1. Anaemia — 50% of patients are anaemic at presentation. This may be caused by marrow infiltration, a Coombs' positive haemolytic anaemia, hypersplenism or, very rarely, red cell aplasia. A positive Coombs' test, caused by a warm IgG antibody, is present in 20% of patients, although only one third of these will develop overt haemolysis. The Coombs' positive haemolytic anaemia may precede the development of other features of chronic lymphatic leukaemia by several years.
2. Thrombocytopenia — this may also be immune, occurring at any stage in the disease. Thrombocytopenia late in the disease is caused by marrow involvement or hypersplenism.
3. Neutropenia — this is rare until the late stages when it is associated with marrow replacement or hypersplenism.

a) Describe the physical signs present. What is the diagnosis?
b) Why is this man in renal failure?
c) Comment on the renal biopsy shown.

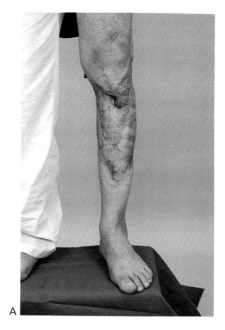

A

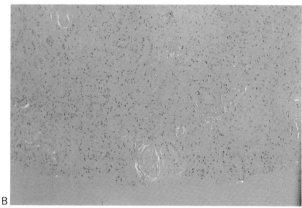

B

a) There is a well demarcated sinus present in the left upper tibia and evidence of previous extensive surgery to the left leg. This man has chronic osteomyelitis of the tibia.

Chronic osteomyelitis may follow an acute osteomyelitis or begin insidiously. The natural history is often one of exacerbations and remissions. Painless discharging sinuses are common. A complete cure is rarely possible.

b) He has developed systemic amyloidosis (AA amyloid) which has caused renal failure. Chronic osteomyelitis may also be complicated by malignant change in the skin around the mouth of the sinus or ulcer.

Systemic amyloidosis is characterized by the deposition of fibrils of AA protein in parenchymal tissue. Clinical features include:

1. Proteinuria, the nephrotic syndrome and renal failure — the cause of death in 50% of cases
2. Hepatosplenomegaly and infiltration of the gut
3. Hypoadrenalism.

AA amyloid is associated with:

1. Chronic infective conditions such as osteomyelitis
2. Chronic inflammatory conditions such as rheumatoid arthritis
3. Chronic malignancies such as Hodgkin's disease and hypernephroma.

c) The renal biopsy has been stained with Congo Red and viewed under polarized light. The classical apple-green uniaxial positive birefringence of amyloid deposition is well seen.

Question 74

a) Slide A: what is the diagnosis?
b) Give a differential diagnosis.
c) Slide B: what investigation has been performed? What does it show and what is the unifying diagnosis for A and B?
d) List the other manifestations of the underlying disease.

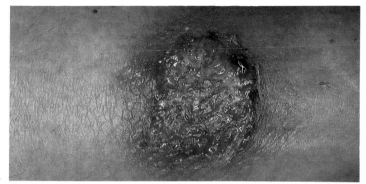

A

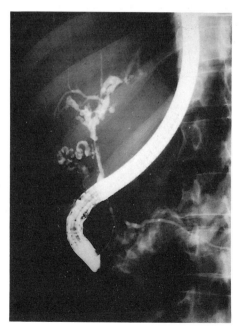

B

a) Pyoderma gangrenosum; there is a large ulcer with a necrotic base and overhanging purple edge.

b) The differential diagnosis includes:

1. Ulcerative colitis
2. Crohn's disease
3. Rheumatoid arthritis
4. Paraproteinaemias
5. Chronic active hepatitis
6. Lymphomas
7. Wegener's granulomatosis.

c) The patient has had an ERCP (endoscopic retrograde cholangiopancreatography) performed which shows the classical appearance of sclerosing cholangitis with narrowing and bead-like dilations of the biliary tree.

Sclerosing cholangitis is characterized by proliferation of scar tissue around intra- and extrahepatic ducts. It occurs in approximately 1% of patients with chronic ulcerative colitis.

d) Ulcerative colitis is a chronic inflammatory condition affecting the mucosa of the colon and rectum. Active disease is associated with fever, bloody diarrhoea, weight loss and anaemia. Local complications of the colitis include: toxic dilatation; severe bleeding; perforation; abscesses and strictures. The risk of developing carcinoma of the colon is increased if the colitis affects the whole colon and is prolonged.

Other features include: anterior uveitis; episcleritis; stomatitis; erythema nodosum; pyoderma gangrenosum; leg ulcers; arthritis; spondylitis, sacroilitis; chronic active hepatitis; cirrhosis; pericholangitis, sclerosing cholangitis; and carcinoma of the biliary tree.

This is the peripheral blood film from a patient with a left radial
nerve palsy. What is the diagnosis?

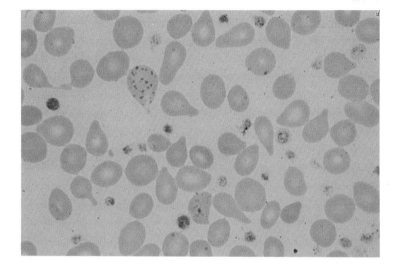

The peripheral red blood cells show basophilic stippling. The coarse (punctate) dots represent condensed RNA in the cytoplasm. In the context of a radial nerve palsy the most likely diagnosis is lead poisoning and does not reflect the severity of the poisoning. It may be absent altogether in severe cases.

Basophilic stippling is also seen in other disorders of haemoglobin synthesis such as pyrimidine-5-nucleotidase deficiency, acquired sideroblastic anaemia and homozygous beta thalassaemias.

The following were noted in a 67-year-old man.
a) What is the ophthalmological diagnosis?
b) Is vision affected?

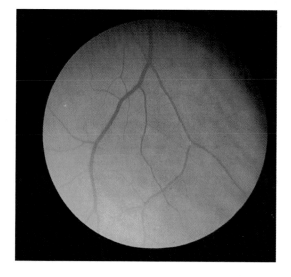

Answer to question 76

a) Hollenhorst plaques, which are cholesterol emboli, are seen here.
b) Vision is usually not affected, since the blood tends to flow around the emboli.

Cholesterol emboli are associated with underlying severe atherosclerotic disease, particularly of the carotids. Angiography, carotid operation, anticoagulation or trauma may precede the embolization of cholesterol crystals. A serious complication of generalized cholesterol embolization is renal involvement, leading to renal failure. Patients may have livedo reticularis as a result of cholesterol emboli lodging in skin vessels.

a) What is the diagnosis?
b) List the recognized associations.
c) What painful complication may occur?

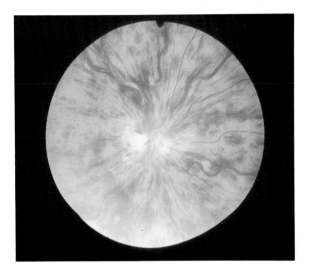

a) Occlusion of the central retinal vein. The slide shows the typical fundal changes which include: venous dilation; widespread haemorrhages, which may be superficial and flame-shaped or deep and blotchy; retinal oedema; cotton wool spots; and swelling of the optic disc.

b) The retinal artery and vein share a common fascial sheath so arteriosclerotic thickening of the artery may result in occlusion of the central retinal vein.

Causes of central retinal vein occlusion include:

1. Hypertension
2. Diabetes mellitus
3. Glaucoma (chronic simple)
4. Hyperviscosity states:
   — Waldenstrom's macroglobulinaemia
   — Polycythaemia rubra vera
   — Less commonly, multiple myeloma.

c) Rubeosis iridis and secondary thrombotic glaucoma. In mild cases recanalization of the central vein may occur with some improvement in vision. In severe cases retinal hypoxia stimulates neovascularization; new vessels develop primarily on the anterior surface of the iris (rubeosis iridis) approximately 90 days after the initial occlusion. Rubeosis iridis may be complicated by thrombotic glaucoma leading to a painful blind eye which may require enucleation.

a) What is the diagnosis in this 16-year-old South American girl?
b) Name the likely organism and vector.
c) What complication may follow?
d) How would you confirm your clinical diagnosis?
e) What drug therapy is appropriate?

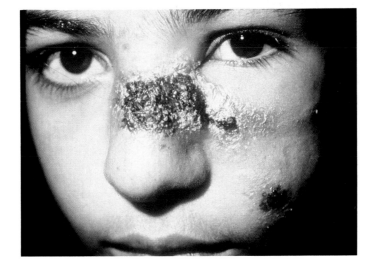

a) Cutaneous leishmaniasis.
b) Leishmaniasis is caused by parasites of the genus *Leishmania*; at
least 12 species cause disease in man. *Leishmania brasiliensis
brasiliensis* is the major cause of American cutaneous
leishmaniasis. The vector is the sand fly; forest rodents are the
likely reservoir of infection.
Leishmania inoculated into the skin by the sand fly bite multiply in
macrophages and cause a nodule which increases in size over
several weeks. The crust often falls off leaving a painless ulcer which
eventually heals leaving a disfiguring scar.
c) Approximately 40% of patients with cutaneous ulcers due to
brasiliensis brasiliensis infection will develop mucocutaneous
leishmaniasis (espundia) with involvement of the nasal mucosa,
pharynx, palate and lip. Untreated mucocutaneous leishmaniasis
tends to slowly progress, eventually destroying the nose and
face.
d) Diagnosis can be confirmed by detecting the parasites in material
obtained from a lesion; the material is smeared, stained (Giemsa
stain) and examined for intracellular parasites. Material is also
inoculated into specific culture media or into hamsters.
The Leishmania skin test is positive in approximately 90% of cases of
cutaneous and mucocutaneous leishmaniasis.
e) Systemic treatment of *brasiliensis brasiliensis* with pentavalent
antimonials, e.g. sodium stibogluconate, is effective and prevents
the disfiguring espudia from developing.

This 45-year-old homeless man was found unconscious and admitted to the accident and emergency department.
a) What clinical sign is seen?
b) What is the underlying diagnosis?
c) Give 3 possible reasons for the loss of consciousness.

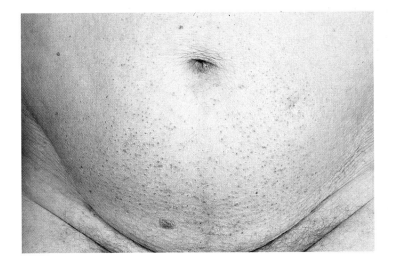

a) Perifollicular haemorrhages.
b) Vitamin C deficiency (scurvy) is the cause. Since citrus fruits and green vegetables are the best source of vitamin C, deficiency is found in some elderly city dwellers living off a diet of tea and toast. Alcoholics are more likely to suffer from B vitamin deficiencies, but vitamin C deficiency is not uncommon in this group. Some patients with chronic diseases such as tuberculosis, smokers and users of oral contraceptives may have low vitamin C levels. The required daily dose is 60 mg, but as little as 10 mg per day is sufficient to prevent scurvy. The body stores are about 1500 mg, and increasing intake dramatically does not substantially increase serum levels or stores. Vitamin C is an anti-oxidant, enhances iron absorption, and is important in collagen hydroxylation. Early symptoms of deficiency are lethargy, followed by bone pain, and later follicular haemorrhage, petechiae, bleeding gums, tooth loss and joint haemorrhage. Intracerebral bleeding may also occur.
c) The following may account for loss of consciousness:

1. Intracerebral bleed due to vitamin C deficiency, or alcoholism
2. Alcoholism, resulting in hypoglycaemia, liver failure, intoxication, vitamin B deficiency, particularly thiamine deficiency, and the Wernicke–Korsakoff syndrome
3. Another drug overdose.

What is the diagnosis?

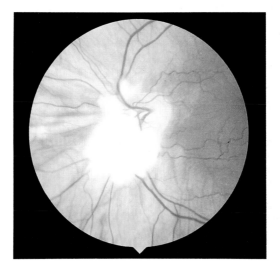

The slide shows the typical flared appearance of medullated nerve fibres which appear brilliantly white in contrast to the red background of the fundus.

The appearance of medullated nerve fibres is due to the presence of myelin sheaths; normally nerve fibres do not have myelin sheaths beyond the lamina cribrosa. The defect is present from birth and is accompanied by a corresponding field defect.

a) What is the diagnosis?
b) List the recognized complications.

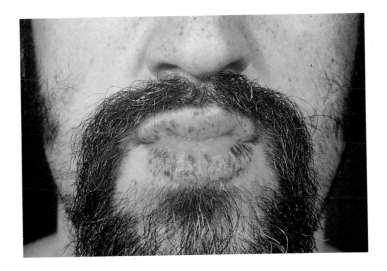

a) This patient has Peutz–Jeghers syndrome; the slide shows typical perioral brown macules extending beyond the margins of the lips.

b) Multiple polyps occur throughout the small intestine and complications include intussusception, anaemia and malignant transformation.

This 40-year-old woman was referred to the vascular surgeons with worsening claudication; she was a non-smoker. Past medical history included myocardial infarction, hypertension and recurrent episodes of upper gastrointestinal blood loss with no evidence of peptic ulceration at endoscopy.

a) What abnormality is present on fundoscopy?

b) What is the diagnosis?

c) What other signs would you look for to confirm your diagnosis?

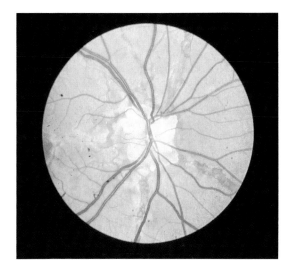

a) The slide shows angioid streaks caused by degeneration of Bruch's membrane – early blindness is common. Common causes of angioid streaks include pseudoxanthoma elasticum, Ehlers–Danlos syndrome, Paget's disease of bone and sickle cell disease. An incidental finding of intrapapillary drusen is also noted.

b) The history of peripheral vascular disease, coronary artery disease, hypertension and gastrointestinal haemorrhage points to a diagnosis of pseudoxanthoma elasticum. Gastrointestinal haemorrhage is a feature of Ehlers–Danlos syndrome but occlusive peripheral and coronary artery disease is not. Pseudoxanthoma elasticum is a hereditary disorder of elastic tissue; four distinct types are recognized, two are autosomal dominant and two autosomal recessive.

c) The skin in pseudoxanthoma elasticum is typically loose, often hanging in folds, and has a chicken skin appearance with small yellow 'pseudoxanthomatous' plaques. Other clinical features of the disease include blue sclerae, myopia, lax joints and mitral valve prolapse.

Note: Intrapapillary drusen are traces of hyaline material seen in 0.4% of Caucasians. The lesions usually progress slowly and are associated with field defects but macula vision is almost never affected.

This 35-year-old man presented with a right femur fracture.
a) What clinical sign is shown?
b) What is the diagnosis?

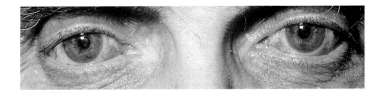

a) Blue sclerae.
b) The combination of blue sclerae and fracture suggests osteogenesis imperfecta.

The differential diagnosis of blue sclerae is:

1. Osteogenesis imperfecta
2. Pseudoxanthoma elasticum
3. Ehlers–Danlos syndrome
4. Marfan's disease
5. Hyperthyroidism.

Osteogenesis imperfecta (OI) is caused by mutations of the Type I collagen gene. Type I collagen is the main collagen component of bone, and consists of a triple helix ($\alpha 1$ and $\alpha 2$ chains). Type I OI is mild, and patients present with blue sclerae, deafness and fractures. Type II OI is the severe infantile form resulting in early death, type III shows short stature due to long bone deformity, grey sclera, and ligamentous laxity, while Type IV is a mild disease. Types I and IV are inherited in an autosomal dominant fashion, while Types II and III are autosomal recessive or sporadic. Treatment is not satisfactory, but maintaining muscle tone with exercise and using orthopaedic devices to prevent deformity and scoliosis are useful. Blue sclerae are usually not seen in Type IV.

Ehlers–Danlos disease consists of 10 different types, with autosomal dominant, recessive, and X-linked recessive inheritance. The abnormalities are in the structure of Type I and III collagen, and progress is being made in unravelling the genetic defects of these diseases. The clinical features vary and include joint hypermobility, skin scarring and stretching, periodontal disease, eye abnormalities such as scleral tears and keratoconus, joint dislocations, arterial and gut rupture. Type IV is associated with the worst prognosis since visceral and arterial rupture is found, but the other types do not adversely affect mortality. Prenatal screening should become possible when more genetic information becomes available, but genetic advice should be sought if a case is identified.

This 45-year-old man presented with a chronic cough and recurrent chest infections requiring antibiotics. On clinical examination he had coarse mid inspiratory crepitations in the right mid zone.

a) What clinical sign is shown and what is the likely cause of the recurrent underlying chest infections?

b) How would you confirm your respiratory diagnosis?

c) How would you manage his chest problem?

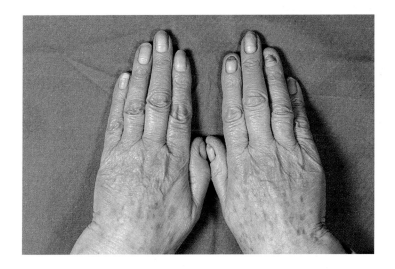

a) Yellow nail syndrome. Shiny yellow nails are associated with abnormal lymphatic drainage. There is an increased incidence of pleural effusions and bronchiectasis. The chest symptoms and signs would be compatible with right mid zone bronchiectasis.
b) CT scan of the thorax.
c) Postural drainage is the key to management combined with courses of antibiotics. Some patients with chronic chest infections require rotating antibiotics. Surgery has a role to play in cases of localized bronchiectasis.

CAUSES OF BRONCHIECTASIS

1. Congenital:
   — Kartagener's syndrome
   — Young's syndrome
   — Cystic fibrosis
   — Primary hypogammaglobulinaemia
2. Acquired:
   — Infections, e.g. TB, measles, whooping cough
   — Benign tumours, e.g. hamartomas.

This young man presented with persistent diarrhoea and weight loss.
a) Slide A: what lesions are shown?
b) Slide B: what organism is visible in this stool specimen?
c) What is the likely underlying diagnosis?

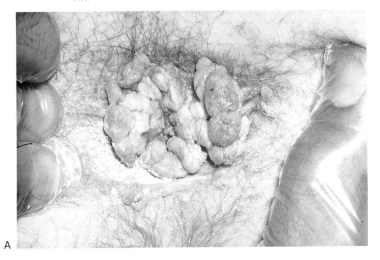

A

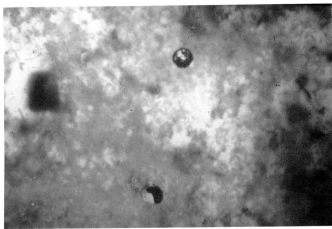

B

a) Anal warts (condylomata accuminata) may be transmitted sexually and occur frequently in homosexual men. They must be distinguished from condylomata lata, a manifestation of secondary syphilis.

b) 'Acid fast' cysts of *Cryptosporidium*, a protozoal parasite widely distributed throughout the animal kingdom. Ziehl–Neelsen staining is useful in identifying the cysts in fresh stool specimens. Cryptosporidium is most easily seen in small bowel biopsies, although the organism may be found throughout the gastrointestinal tract.

Clinical features of cryptosporidium infection include:

1. Diarrhoea, which may be severe in immunocompromised patients
2. Variable villous atrophy
3. Malabsorption.

Cryptosporidium is the commonest pathogen isolated from AIDS patients with diarrhoea.

No treatment is necessary in immunocompetent individuals who generally have a mild self-limiting illness. Spiramycin may be effective in controlling the infection in immunocompromised individuals.

c) AIDS — the combination of anal warts and cryptosporidium.

a) What is the diagnosis?
b) What are the two commonest associations?

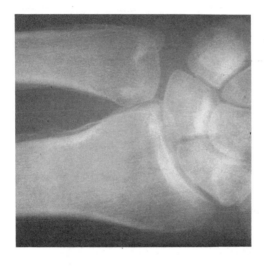

a) Hypertrophic pulmonary osteoarthropathy (HPOA). The slide shows subperiosteal new bone formation along the diaphyses of the radius and ulna; similar changes may be seen in the tibia and fibula. HPOA is often accompanied by clubbing and an arthritis affecting the wrists and ankles.

b) Hypertrophic pulmonary osteoarthropathy is most commonly associated with squamous carcinoma of the lung and pleural mesothelioma.

Rarely it may accompany pleural fibromas, intrapulmonary sepsis, cyanotic congenital heart disease and β-hCG secreting tumours such as teratomas or trophoblastic tumours. HPOA associated with tumours may be accompanied by gynaecomastia.

a) Describe the abnormalities present.
b) The patient's mother and brother are similarly affected; what is the most likely diagnosis?

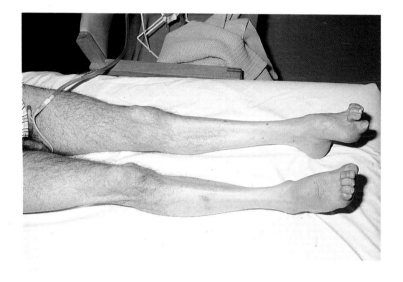

a) There is distal muscle wasting which stops around mid thigh —
'inverted champagne bottles'. The toes are clawed and there is a
pes cavus deformity. There is a urinary catheter in place.

b) The differential diagnosis of pes cavus and muscle wasting
includes:

1. Charcot–Marie–Tooth disease
2. Old polio infection
3. Friedreich's ataxia
4. Spina bifida.

In this case the family history and symmetrical pattern of muscle
wasting suggests a diagnosis of Charcot–Marie–Tooth disease
(peroneal muscular atrophy/hereditary motor and sensory
neuropathy). The urinary catheter is incidental.

Other clinical features include: a characteristic 'steppage gait' due
to the bilateral foot drop; wasting of the small muscles of the hand;
thickened peripheral nerves; areflexia; distal sensory neuropathy;
digital trophic ulceration; upper limb tremor; and scoliosis.

Charcot–Marie–Tooth disease is inherited in an autosomal
dominant manner with variable penetrance. Two types of peroneal
muscular atrophy may be distinguished.

Type I is commoner, has an earlier age of onset (first decade) and
is associated with more severe clinical features than Type II.
Peripheral nerve thickening, diffuse demyelination and reduced nerve
conduction velocities are features of Type I and not Type II.

Cases associated with ataxia have been described and are referred
to as the Roussy–Levy syndrome.

What complication has arisen in this bone marrow transplant recipient?

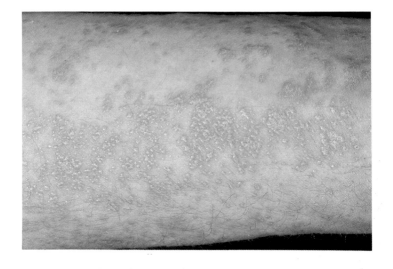

The patient has developed lichen planus. The slide shows typical flat-topped purple polygonal papules. Lichen planus usually starts on the flexor aspect of the wrist; lesions on the shins may coalesce forming hypertrophic plaques. The fine, white, lace-like lesions visible on the surface of some papules are called Wickham's striae. Mucosal lesions occur in up to 70% of cases; they are usually visible opposite the premolar teeth, in severe cases ulceration can occur. Lichen planus, along with psoriasis and viral warts, exhibits the Koebner phenomenon (further lesions develop at sites of trauma).

Histology of lichen planus lesions shows a heavy lymphocytic infiltrate adjacent to the lower surface of the epidermis, liquefactive degeneration of the epidermal basement membrane and saw toothing of the rete ridges. Other features include hyperkeratosis and an increase in the epidermal granular layer. Pathogenesis is poorly understood, although an immunological mechanism seems likely. Recognized causes of lichen planus include:

1. Graft versus host disease following bone marrow transplant
2. Drugs, e.g. gold, penicillamine, antimalarials, sulphonylureas, beta blockers, thiazides, methyldopa
3. Chemicals (e.g. colour developers).

Topical steroids, often in combination with polythene occlusion, are the treatment of choice for mild cases; oral steroids are used in severe cases. Metronidazole is effective for ulcerative oral lichen planus.

This is the peripheral blood from a 69-year-old woman who presented with tiredness. Her full blood count was Hb 9.8 g/dl, MCV 104 fl, WBC 5.6 × 10⁹/l, Plts 138 × 10⁹/l.
What is the likely diagnosis?

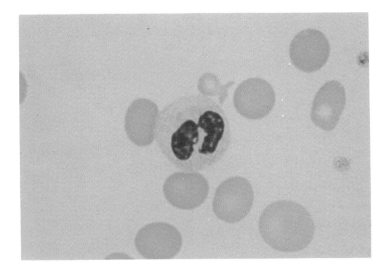

Answer to question 89

The blood film shows a Pelger–Huet neutrophil with characteristic hypogranular cytoplasm and bilobed nucleus.

Pelger–Huet neutrophils can be inherited as part of a rare autosomal dominant trait but are more commonly seen in myelodysplastic syndromes. Pelger cells may antedate other features of myelodysplasia by months or years.

The myelodysplastic syndromes are clonal disorders of haemopoietic stem cells and are characterized by peripheral blood cytopenias and abnormalities of erythroid, myeloid or megakaryocyte development in the bone marrow; they are associated with a very high risk of leukaemic transformation.

Myelodysplasia tends to develop in older patients but is also seen in younger patients who have received intensive chemotherapy for other haematological malignancies or solid tumours.

a) What is the diagnosis?
b) What factors predispose patients to this condition?

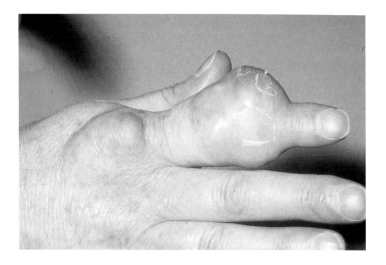

a) Chronic tophaceous gout. Gout progresses from hyperuricaemia to regular attacks of acute gout and, if left untreated, after an average of twelve years to chronic tophaceous gout. This stage is characterized by:

1. Tophi: chalky deposits containing urate crystals which may occur anywhere but are most commonly found on the ears, hands, around affected joints and occasionally in bursae
2. Gouty joint erosions which are juxta-articular and generally large.

The rate of formation of tophi is a function of the degree and duration of the hyperuricaemia. As tophi and urate-induced renal disease advance, acute attacks of gout occur less frequently. The tophi themselves are not painful but do cause deformity which may be crippling. Complications of the tophi include ulceration, infection and rarely bony ankylosis. Tophi may occur in the myocardium, mitral valve, cardiac conduction system, eye, larynx, and may even cause spinal compression.

b) Conditions which lead to hyperuricaemia and may eventually lead to tophi include:

1. Primary gout, either 'over-producers' or 'under-secretors' of urate
2. Drugs, e.g. diuretics, ethambutol, pyrazinamide
3. Myeloproliferative disorders, especially polycythaemia rubra vera, chronic haemolytic anaemias and severe skin disease (increased turnover of nucleic acids)
4. Renal disease, a rare cause of gout
5. Lead poisoning
6. Hyperparathyroidism and hypothyroidism decreasing renal tubule urate excretion
7. Inherited enzyme defects, including Lesch–Nyhan syndrome, an inherited deficiency of hypoxanthine-guanine phosphoribosyl transferase
8. Glycogen storage disease Type 1.

This young Caucasian girl has a deep voice and a blood pressure of 180/105.
a) What physical signs are present?
b) What diagnostic procedure has been performed? What is the diagnosis?
c) What other physical signs would you expect to find and how can you account for them?

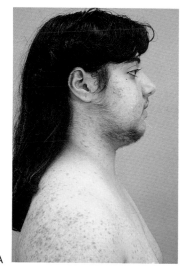

A

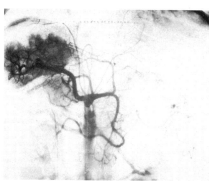

B

a) The slide shows a girl who is Cushingoid and hirsute. The male pattern of facial hair and the deep voice indicate virilization.

b) The angiogram shows a large well vascularized lesion adjacent to the right kidney, consistent with an adrenal carcinoma.

c) Other clinical indications of virilization which might be present include: clitoromegaly; loss of libido; and increased skin thickness. Excess cortisol production by the tumour accounts for her Cushingoid appearance and hypertension.

Adrenal carcinoma is a rare disease whose features depend on the patient's sex and the biologically active steroids secreted. Males may present with precocious puberty and/or Cushing's syndrome.

If there is no steroid production, patients may present with an abdominal mass, or symptoms related to secondary deposits.

Elevated blood and urine levels of dehydroepiandrosterone (DHAE), testosterone, 11-deoxycortisol and cortisol may be found. Urinary 17-oxo or 17-oxogeneic steroids are usually greatly raised.

Diagnosis depends on radiological identification of the tumour using ultrasound, CT scanning and angiography.

Differential diagnosis of virilization in a female includes:

1. Congenital adrenal hyperplasia
2. Androgen-secreting ovarian neoplasm
3. Androgen-secreting adrenal adenoma
4. Polycystic ovaries.

Surgical removal of the tumour should be attempted, although it is rarely complete due to local invasion of the renal vein and surrounding tissues. Steroid supplements are often necessary post surgery as the cortisol-secreting neoplasm suppresses ACTH production which results in atrophy of normal adrenal tissue. Late metastases are common. Androgen levels are a useful means of detecting recurrence.

This man's father died at the age of 35.
a) What is the echocardiographic diagnosis?
b) How does the condition usually manifest itself and what are the recognized clinical signs?

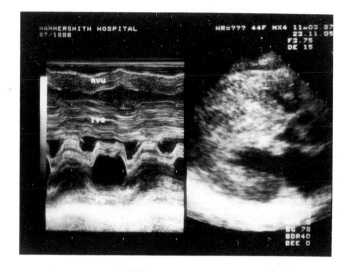

a) This slide shows a parasternal long axis view (right) and the M mode recording (left) from a patient with hypertrophic obstructive cardiomyopathy (HOCM). There is disproportional (asymmetric) septal hypertrophy (3–4 cm), poor systolic thickening of the septum and a systolic anterior motion of the mitral valve (SAM). Note also that the right ventricular wall is hypertrophied.
IVS = intraventricular septum, RVW = right ventricular wall.

b) Hypertrophic obstructive cardiomyopathy (HOCM) is inherited as an autosomal dominant trait, although sporadic cases occur. HOCM often presents in the second decade with shortness of breath resulting from an elevated left atrial pressure. Other presentations include syncope, angina and palpitations (atrial and ventricular arrhythmias are common).
Clinical signs include:

1. A jerky but sustained pulse with a rapid initial upstroke followed by a sustained component
2. A double apical impulse composed of a palpable atrial beat followed by the prominent left ventricular impulse
3. III and IV heart sounds
4. A late systolic apical murmur whose intensity is diminished by squatting or isometric hand exercises and increased by amylnitrate or the Valsalva manoeuvre.

Currently the detection and treatment of ventricular arrhythmias appears to provide the best approach to reducing the risk of sudden death. Amiodarone is the drug of choice for arrhythmia prophylaxis.

Question 93

This is the peripheral blood from a 25-year-old diplomat with fever. What is the diagnosis?

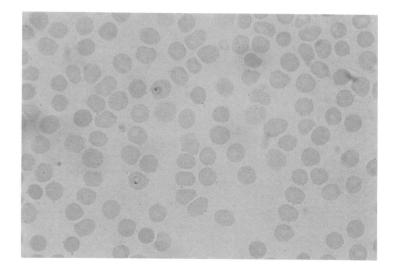

There are numerous ring forms and the diagnosis is *Plasmodium falciparum* malaria. Parasitaemia greater than 0.5% usually indicates falciparum malaria. Note the absence of platelets on the blood film.

Thrombocytopenia is very common in both falciparum and vivax malaria. Malaria must be excluded in any patient with fever who has returned from a malarious zone. There is increasing chloroquine resistance worldwide and a detailed travel history is critical. If the patient comes from an area where chloroquine resistance has been documented or is suspected, treatment with quinine should be commenced as soon as possible. Quinine therapy may produce cinchonism — tinnitus, giddiness, tremulousness and blurred vision. Hypoglycaemia may be a feature of severe falciparum malaria and can complicate quinine treatment. Quinine can rarely cause arrhythmias and thrombocytopenia.

This 25-year-old man has reacted adversely to the sunlight from childhood, developing widespread erythema and swelling up to 72 hours after exposure.
  What is the diagnosis?

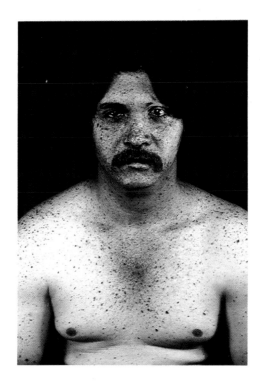

.The patient has xeroderma pigmentosa.

Xeroderma pigmentosa, inherited in an autosomal recessive fashion, is caused by deficiency of a DNA repair enzyme normally responsible for the repair of DNA damaged by ultraviolet light. The first signs, which occur in infancy, are marked erythema and cutaneous swelling up to 72 hours after exposure to sunlight. After further damage there is patchy macular pigmentation, multiple keratoses and telangiectasia. There is an increase in basal cell carcinomas, squamous cell carcinomas and malignant melanomas.

This 26-year-old female on return from Kenya developed a fever and
a macular rash. She was also noted to have the lesion shown.
a) What is the most likely diagnosis?
b) How would you confirm your diagnosis?
c) What treatment would you give?

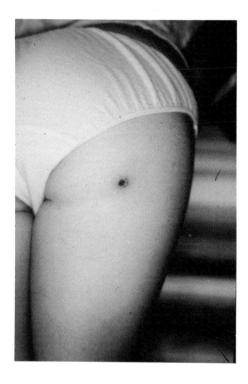

a) The slide shows a tick eschar. The most likely diagnosis is tick-borne typhus, an illness caused by *Rickettsia conori* (fièvre boutonneuse) which is distributed throughout the Mediterranean, India and Africa.

Tick typhus is one of the spotted fever group of rickettsial diseases which include Rocky Mountain spotted fever and Q fever.

Rickettsiae are obligate intracellular parasites. Most rickettsiae are adapted to a cycle involving an insect vector and an animal reservoir, man being an accidental sporadic victim.

An eschar develops at the site of the tick bite in 50% of cases. The organisms invade endothelial cells throughout the body causing vasculitis and thrombotic occlusion with subsequent necrosis.

All the rickettsial illnesses follow a similar pattern, though the severity varies. Rocky Mountain spotted fever, the paradigm, is the most severe. The illness is characterized by fever (lasting one to two weeks), headache, photophobia, profound malaise, a haemorrhagic or maculopapular rash which begins peripherally, lymphadenopathy, hepatosplenomegaly and central nervous system involvement. Cardiovascular failure, liver failure and renal failure may complicate severe infection.

The history of travel to an endemic area and the presence of a tick eschar are helpful in making a diagnosis.

b) The diagnosis is confirmed serologically.

1. The Weil–Felix reaction detects antibodies which cause agglutination of *Proteus* OX 19 strains. It is positive in a number of rickettsial illnesses and false positive results occur with a number of other fevers.
2. Specific serological tests are available for all of the major rickettsioses.

c) Chloramphenicol or tetracycline are the antibiotics of choice.

a) What is this physical sign?
b) With what conditions is this sign associated?

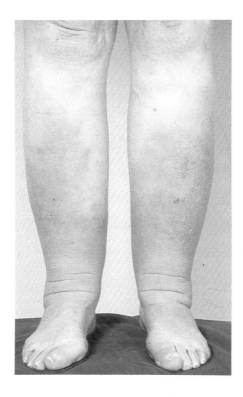

a) Pre-tibial myxoedema. The slide shows red-brown, thickened skin with a peau d'orange appearance.

b) Graves' disease, ophthalmic Graves' disease and thyroid acropachy are all associated with pre-tibial myxoedema. As with ophthalmic Graves' disease, pre-tibial myxoedema may be found in the absence of other features of autoimmune thyroid disease, and can appear after treatment of hyperthyroidism in Graves' disease.

Biopsy of areas of pre-tibial myxoedema is not recommended as lesions heal slowly, often with keloid formation. Histology of affected skin shows infiltration of the subcutaneous tissue with glycosaminoglycans.

Deposits tend to persist despite biochemical control of hyperthyroidism; treatment with topical steroids may be effective.

This 7-year-old boy, pictured here with his brother, was unable to play football.
a) What sign is illustrated?
b) What is the diagnosis?

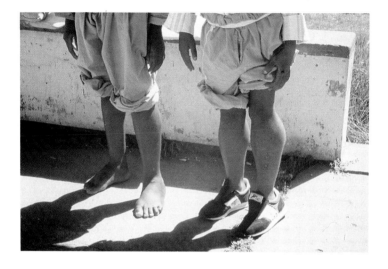

a) Pseudohypertrophy of the calf muscles.
b) Duchenne's muscular dystrophy is usually inherited in an X-linked recessive manner. However up to 30% arise by spontaneous mutation. The disease affects 30 per 100 000 live male births and is the commonest and most serious of the muscular dystrophies. Female carriers remain asymptomatic but may have high levels of creatinine kinase. Symptoms of muscle weakness usually appear by 5 years of age and include a lordotic waddling gait, frequent falls and difficulty climbing stairs. Pseudohypertrophy of the calves is an early sign. Although the muscles are large they are also weak; later there is severe muscle wasting. When affected individuals rise from lying they characteristically 'climb up their knees' — this is Gower's sign. Most patients are wheelchair bound by 10 years of age; scoliosis and equinus foot deformities are common. Cardiomyopathy is also a common feature. Death usually occurs in the early twenties following a respiratory tract infection.

The diagnosis is confirmed by:

1. Elevated levels of serum creatinine kinase
2. Myopathic changes on the electromyelogram
3. Muscle biopsy findings — variation in fibre size with internal nuclei and fibre degeneration.

Becker muscular dystrophy (X-linked recessive) is similar in nature to Duchenne's muscular dystrophy but is milder in form and has a later age of onset in the mid twenties.

The lesions on this man's foot have developed slowly and are now painful and itchy.
a) What is the diagnosis?
b) How would you confirm your diagnosis?

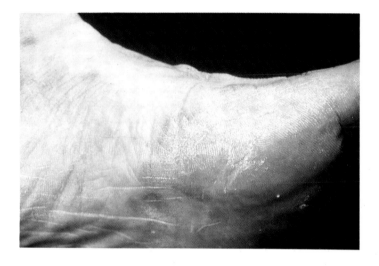

a) The lesions are Kaposi's sarcomas.
b) The foot lesions should be biopsied to confirm the diagnosis.

Serological evidence of human immunodeficiency virus (HIV) infection should be sought after counselling the patient. Kaposi's sarcoma is the commonest malignancy seen in association with the acquired immune deficiency syndrome (AIDS). Prior to the AIDS epidemic two distinct patterns of Kaposi's sarcoma were recognized:

1. A nodular localized malignancy, typically on the lower extremities, occurring in elderly men of Jewish or Mediterranean descent
2. A rapidly progressive malignancy seen in young African children.

Kaposi's sarcoma is seen in between 14% and 21% of homosexual AIDS patients but is rare in HIV infected drug abusers or haemophiliacs. The lesions begin as violaceous papules which first darken like a bruise and later become raised firm nodules, which may be painful. They may occur in several sites simultaneously. The skin lesions are however frequently atypical, therefore any suspicious lesion should be biopsied. AIDS related Kaposi's disseminates to local lymph nodes, the gastrointestinal tract, the central nervous system, lung, liver, spleen and testes.

Chemotherapy with vinblastine is useful for early disease; late or aggressive disease can be treated with combination regimens including α-interferon.

Radiotherapy may be used for skin lesions, pulmonary lesions and lymphadenopathy which is causing pressure symptoms.

Question 99

a) What is the diagnosis?
b) List the recognized related cardiovascular abnormalities.
c) How is the condition inherited?

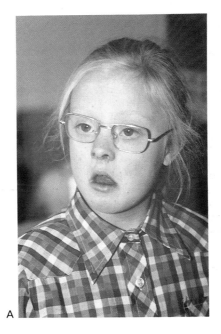

A

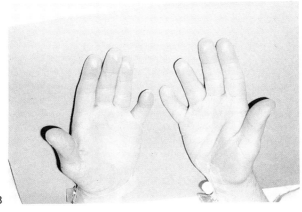

B

a) Down's syndrome — trisomy 21.
   Slide A shows the typical oval face with prominent epicanthic folds and large tongue.
   Slide B shows the characteristic incurving little finger.
   Other phenotypic abnormalities include: mental retardation; general hypotonia; brachycephaly; short stature; Brushfield spots; cataracts; transverse palmar crease; dermatoglyphic abnormalities; strabismus; and nystagmus.

b) Cardiovascular abnormalities occur in approximately 40% of patients. They include atrial septal defect, ventricular septal defect, Fallot's tetralogy and patent ductus arteriosus.
Other recognized associations of Down's syndrome are: duodenal atresia; imperforate anus; hypothyroidism; and male infertility. A decline in IQ in late childhood is often associated with the development of a syndrome similar to Alzheimer's disease. The incidence of leukaemia in Down's syndrome is 10–18 times that in the normal population.

c) Down's syndrome usually arises from non-dysjunction of chromosomes 21 during meiosis. The risk of a Down's child is 1:1000 for women between 20 and 29 years of age but rises to 1:60 for women over 40. A couple with one Down's child due to non-dysjunction run an overall risk of 1:100 of having a second Down's baby. Approximately 6% arise by Robertsonian translocation, usually involving chromosomes 14 and 21. A woman carrying such a translocation has a 1:8 risk of a Down's baby and a father a 1:50 chance. 2% of cases are associated with mosaicism which arises by mitotic non-dysjunction after formation of the zygote. Mosaics may have a normal IQ but tend to bear the physical stigmata of the syndrome, the greater the number of cells carrying the trisomy the greater the abnormality.

This 25-year-old actor presented to rheumatology outpatients with a swollen right knee and a painful left third toe.
a) What sign is shown?
b) What is the likely diagnosis?
c) List the other clinical features.

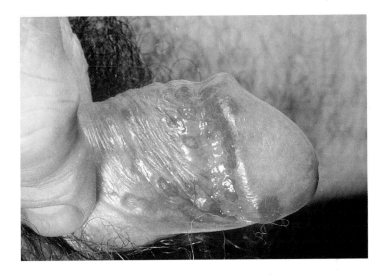

a) The typical appearance of circinate balanitis is well shown. Painless vesicles first appear on the coronal margin of the prepuce and adjacent glans and later they rupture to form superficial erosions which may coalesce to form the typical circinate pattern.

b) Reiter's syndrome. This reactive arthropathy is typically seen in patients between the ages of 16 and 35 years. Two distinct types of reactive arthritis are recognized, one complicating urethral tract infections with mycoplasma or chlamydia, and the other following episodes of dysentery with salmonella, shigella, yersinia and campylobacter. Post-venereal reactive arthritis is much commoner in males than females and there is a strong genetic association with HLA B27. Recurrent or chronic disease occurs in up to 60% of patients.

c) Clinical features:

1. Musculoskeletal
   — Acute asymmetrical oligoarthritis affecting large and small joints, typically of the lower limb, though upper limb involvement is described
   — Enthesopathy is common, e.g. Achilles tendonitis, plantar fasciitis
   — Sacroiliitis occurs in up to 33%
2. Ocular
   — Conjunctivitis
   — Iritis
3. Cutaneous
   — Circinate balantitis (20–50%)
   — Keratoderma blenorrhagica — yellow waxy warty lesions on the soles of the feet occur in up to 15% of patients
   — Painless oral aphthous ulceration occurs in up to 10% of patients
   — Dystrophic nails
4. Systemic disturbance — malaise, fever.

Rare but recognized features of chronic disease include cardiac conduction defects, aortic regurgitation, pericarditis, pulmonary infiltrates and peripheral neuropathy.

This is the peripheral blood film and bone marrow from a 55-year-old patient with acute renal failure.

a) What abnormalities are present on the peripheral blood film?

b) What diagnosis is confirmed by the bone marrow aspirate?

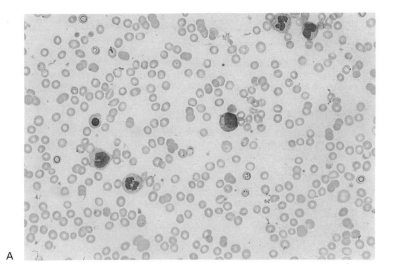

A

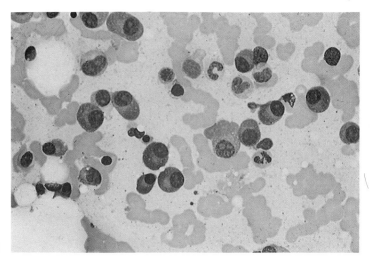

B

a) The peripheral blood film shows nucleated red blood cells and myelocytes — a leukoerythroblastic blood picture. Rouleaux are also present. A leukoerythroblastic blood film with prominent rouleaux formation in a patient with renal failure is highly suggestive of multiple myeloma.

b) The diagnosis of multiple myeloma is confirmed by the plasma cell infiltrate seen in the marrow aspirate. Plasma cells are characterized by their prominent basophilic cytoplasm, eccentric nucleus and perinuclear halo.

A leukoerythroblastic blood film is caused by disruption of normal bone marrow architecture, either by accumulation of abnormal cells or by marrow fibrosis. It may also be seen in conditions of severe marrow stress, such as haemolysis. Bone marrow examination is essential unless a readily reversible factor is identified. The underlying disorder is often only demonstrated by a bone marrow trephine since the bone marrow aspirate is often dry when there is marrow infiltration.

The common causes of a leukoerythroblastic blood film include:

1. Bone marrow infiltration
   — Metastatic carcinoma
   — Multiple myeloma
   — Leukaemia
   — Lymphoma
   — Myelosclerosis
2. Stressed marrow
   — Haemolysis
   — Hypoxia.

Renal impairment is present in approximately 50% of patients at the time of presentation and often has a complex aetiology. Histologically the two commonest findings are: myeloma cast nephropathy in which dense obstructive casts cause tubular obstruction and a consequent interstitial nephritis; and a glomerular lesion caused by the deposition of amyloid and light chains. Other factors which contribute to renal impairment include:

1. Hypovolaemia
2. Hypercalcaemia
3. Hyperuricaemia
4. Administration of radio-iodine contrast media to a patient with myeloma and compromised renal function or marginal hypovolaemia is especially hazardous.

This man complains of low back pain and his general practitioner has documented glycosuria in the presence of a normal blood glucose level.

a) What is the diagnosis?

b) How do you explain the glycosuria?

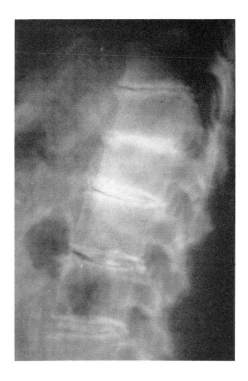

a) Alkaptonuria (ochronosis). Alkaptonuria is an autosomal recessive deficiency of the enzyme homogentisic acid oxidase, which results in excess homogentisic acid accumulating in the blood, tissues and urine. Oxidation and polymerization of homogentisic acid leads to the deposition of a black pigment alkapton in the connective tissue of the joints, intervertebral discs, sclerae, ears, nose, trachea and large vessels. The majority of patients present in middle age with back pain and stiffness. Degenerative arthritis of the knees, hips and shoulders is also common. The condition is compatible with a normal life span and treatment is aimed at relieving symptoms.
Alkapton deposition in the ears and eyes aids the diagnosis. The urine will turn dark on standing, however the change is often protracted unless the process is speeded up by alkalinization of the urine. Urine chromatography confirms the diagnosis.
   The slide shows narrowed, calcified intervertebral discs with minimal osteophyte formation; NB the interspinous ligament does not calcify and the sacroiliac joints are unaffected.

b) The reported glycosuria is a false positive Clinitest result. Homogentisic acid is a reducing substance and as such, like all reducing substances, will give a positive result with Clinitest tablets; it will not however give a positive reaction with Clinistix. Clinistix contains the enzyme glucose oxidase and is specific for glucose.

This young man presented with heel pain and a stiff back.
a) What investigation has been performed?
b) What does it show?
c) Suggest a likely diagnosis?

anterior chest anterior pelvis

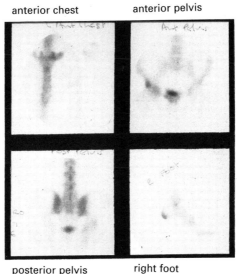

posterior pelvis right foot

a) A bone scan.
b) Hot spots are visible over both sacroiliac joints and the right heel.
c) The most likely diagnosis is ankylosing spondylitis.

Ankylosing spondylitis is the most likely diagnosis in a young man with bilateral sacroiliitis and plantar fasciitis. Ankylosing spondylitis is characterized by sacroiliitis, spondylitis, inflammation of entheses and peripheral arthritis (hips, knees, shoulders and wrists). Males are affected twice as commonly as females. The MHC antigen HLA B27 is found in 96% of Caucasian cases.

  Sacroiliac joints are usually the first joints affected, the patient presenting with low back pain and early morning stiffness. Radiologically sacroiliitis, which is usually symmetrical, is the hallmark of the disease. Bone scans will reveal sacroiliac inflammation before changes are visible on the plain X-ray. Involvement of the lumbar and thoracic spine follows. Erosion of the upper anterior corner of the vertebral body is the earliest radiological sign of spinal disease (the Romanus lesion); subsequent calcification causes squaring of the lumbar vertebrae. Calcification of the annulus fibrosus forms syndesmophytes, and calcification of the interspinous ligaments and longitudinal ligaments produces the typical 'bamboo spine' appearance. Restriction of chest expansion less than 2.5 cm is common in advanced cases.

  Enthesitis leads to erosions and subsequent soft tissue calcification, e.g. plantar spur, calcification of the ischial tuberosities and iliac crest.

Associated features of ankylosing spondylitis include:

1. Asymptomatic prostatitis (80%)
2. Anterior uveitis (25%) and conjunctivitis (20%)
3. Cardiac conduction defects, aortic incompetence
4. Pulmonary fibrosis — typically apical
5. Amyloidosis
6. Cauda equina syndrome

Note: An enthesis is the point of insertion of a capsule, ligament or tendon into bone.

a) What is the diagnosis?
b) Give a differential diagnosis?

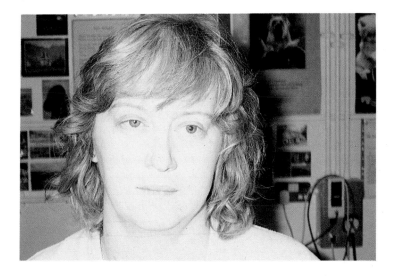

a) The patient has a right Horner's syndrome: ipsilateral ptosis and meiosis (smaller pupil). Associated features include enophthalmos, impaired sweating over the forehead, a blocked nose and a bloodshot cornea. This patient developed Horner's syndrome as a complication of a right internal jugular line insertion, the scar of which is visible.

b) Horner's syndrome results from any lesion interrupting the sympathetic supply to the eye. There are three neurones involved: the first passes from the hypothalamus to the lateral grey matter in the thoracic cord; the second from the cord, via the T1 root, to the superior cervical ganglion; the third, from the superior cervical ganglion, follows the carotid artery to join the long ciliary and third cranial nerves to supply the pupil and levator palpebrae superioris.

Causes of Horner's syndrome include:

1. Hypothalamic lesions
2. Brain stem lesions, e.g. lateral medullary syndrome
3. Cervical cord lesions, e.g. syringomyelia
4. Lesions affecting T1 spinal root, e.g. Pancoast tumour
5. Lesions affecting the sympathetic chain, e.g. surgery, trauma, neoplasm.

Question 105

a) Slide A — what is the diagnosis?
b) Slide B — what is the diagnosis?

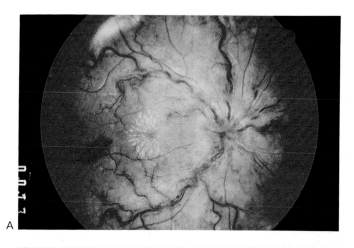

A

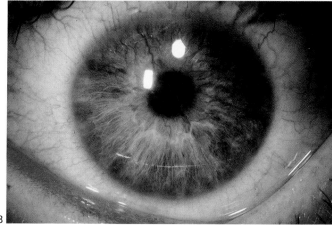

B

a) Grade 4 accelerated phase hypertension. The slide shows papilloedema, widespread haemorrhages, cotton wool spots and a macula star.
Hypertensive retinopathy may be graded:

Grade 1: Arterial constriction and heightened light reflex (copper/silver wiring)
Grade 2: Arterial venous nipping
Grade 3: Haemorrhages, cotton wool spots and hard exudates (macula star)
Grade 4: Papilloedema.

b) Rubeosis iridis. The slide shows new vessel formation on the iris, a response to ischaemia. Rubeosis is a recognized complication of diabetes and retinal vein occlusion.

a) What clinical sign is shown?
b) What is the underlying diagnosis?
c) What are the recognized associated features?

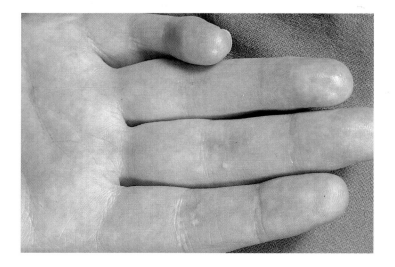

a) Palmar xanthomata.
b) Type III hyperlipoproteinaemia (broad-beta disease).
Type III hyperlipidaemia occurs in 1:5000 individuals and is characterized by high circulating levels of IDL (intermediate density lipoproteins) leading to high serum cholesterol and triglyceride levels. It is generally thought to be an autosomal recessive condition due to a mutation or polymorphism affecting the apoE gene. It is rare in premenopausal women because oestrogens enhance hepatic uptake of IDL. Striate palmar xanthomata are present in 50% of individuals and typically take the form of orange-yellow seed-like lesions within the palmar and finger creases.
c) Tuboeruptive xanthomata — yellow nodular lesions over the tuberosities — are also seen. Accelerated atherosclerosis of the femoral and tibial arteries leading to vascular claudication and premature coronary disease is typically seen.

This 35-year-old businessman returned six weeks ago from a holiday in Thailand. He is generally well. On examination, there is widespread lymphadenopathy and the palmar rash shown.
a) What is the probable diagnosis?
b) List four other clinical features which might be present.
c) How is the diagnosis confirmed?
d) What treatment would you advise?

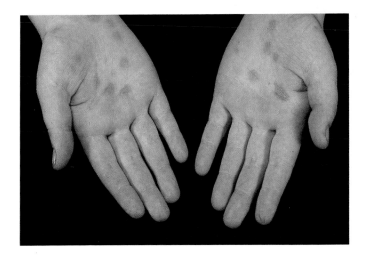

a) Secondary syphilis. The slide shows symmetrical, well demarcated, dusky red palmar lesions typical of secondary syphilis.

The lesions of secondary syphilis occur 4–8 weeks after the primary lesion (chancre), which may still be present in up to a third of cases.

Clinical manifestations vary greatly. Some patients present with malaise and a widespread symmetrical macular or maculopapular, non-itchy rash (lesions crop, collarettes are present). Others present with a subtle transient eruption over the flanks. Widespread discrete non-tender lymphadenopathy is common.

b) Other clinical manifestations of secondary syphilis include:

1. Shallow, painless erosions of mucous membranes — snail track ulcers
2. Condylomata lata; in warm moist areas papular lesions may coalesce to form large fleshy masses
3. Alopecia
4. Eye — uveitis, choroidoretinitis, optic neuritis
5. Locomotor — arthritis, periostitis
6. Neurological — meningitis, cranial nerve palsies.

Rarely — hepatitis, glomerulonephritis and the nephrotic syndrome.

c) The diagnosis of syphilis may be confirmed by:

1. Dark field microscopy, using material from the chancre or lymph nodes to demonstrate the spiral, motile *Treponema pallidum* organisms
2. Serology: serological tests only become positive 5–8 weeks after the original infection.

- Non-specific tests: VDRL flocculation test. Treponemal diseases including yaws, pinta and bejel will also yield positive reactions. Biological false positives are common (leprosy, connective tissue diseases) and false negatives may occur.
- Specific tests: Fluorescent treponemal antibody test (FTA); *Treponema pallidum* haemagglutination assay (TPHA).

d) 600 mg of procaine penicillin intramuscularly for 10 days. In cases of penicillin allergy alternatives include tetracycline or erythromycin. A mild Jarish–Herxheimer reaction commonly complicates treatment of secondary syphilis. This reaction (fever, tachycardia, vasodilation and a flare of the existing rash) is believed to be due to release of endotoxin from the large number of organisms killed by the penicillin.

This man presents with diarrhoea and loss of weight.
a) What clinical sign is present?
b) What is this appearance due to?
c) List two predisposing factors.

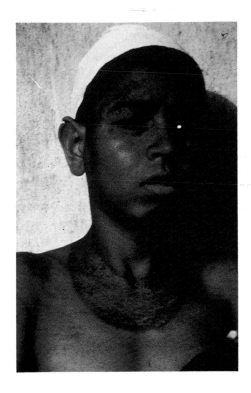

a) The slide shows the classic appearance of Casal's necklace — a photosensitive dermatitis prominent over the neck and upper chest.

b) Niacin (nicotinamide) deficiency. The deficiency state is called pellagra and is characterized by loss of appetite, weakness, glossitis and the triad of diarrhoea, dementia and dermatitis. The dermatitis is most marked in light exposed areas. Erythema and pruritus are followed by flaking, pigmentation and finally fissuring. Niacin as NAD or NADP is an important co-factor in cellular oxidation–reduction reactions.

c) Niacin is available in a wide variety of foods, and body requirements are supplemented by niacin synthesis from tryptophan.

Niacin deficiency is likely to occur when maize forms a large part of the dietary intake as maize is low in both niacin and tryptophan. Two other situations which predispose to niacin deficiency are carcinoid syndrome (the tumour converts tryptophan to 5-hydroxytryptamine) and Hartnup disease (tryptophan is poorly absorbed).

In pellagra, niacin metabolites, e.g. urinary N-methylnicotinamide, are undetectable and fasting plasma tryptophan concentrations are low.

Untreated pellagra has a substantial mortality; treatment takes the form of niacin supplements.

This man presented at the age of 12 with haemolytic anaemia.
a) What clinical sign is shown?
b) What is the diagnosis?
c) What are the other recognized features of this condition?

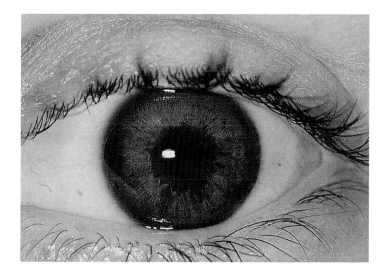

a) A Kayser–Fleischer ring. The typical appearance of copper
deposition in the limbus of the cornea is shown.
b) Wilson's disease, an autosomal recessive disorder due to
mutation of a gene on the long arm of chromosome 13. It is
characterized by absent or greatly reduced caeruloplasmin
plasma levels but the pathogenetic abnormality is a reduction in
the biliary excretion of copper. Tissue levels of copper are high,
especially in the liver, brain, cornea and kidney.
c) Clinical features include:

1. Haematological — Coombs' negative haemolysis 10%
2. Hepatic
   — Hepatitis
   — Cirrhosis with portal hypertension; rarely may present with
     fulminant hepatic failure
   — Pigment gall stones due to haemolysis
3. Neurological
   — Behavioural problems
   — Parkinsonian features
4. Renal — proximal renal tubular acidosis
5. Ocular — Kayser–Fleischer ring
6. Musculoskeletal — early osteoarthritis
7. Nails — blue nails.

Diagnosis is made by demonstrating low plasma caeruloplasmin
levels. Plasma copper may be normal or low (increased free copper),
but urine copper levels are high.
   Treatment includes a low copper diet, copper chelation with
penicillamine, trientine or oral zinc (may prevent copper absorption).

This man presented with interscapular pain.
a) What is the echocardiographic diagnosis?
b) What are the recognized predisposing factors?

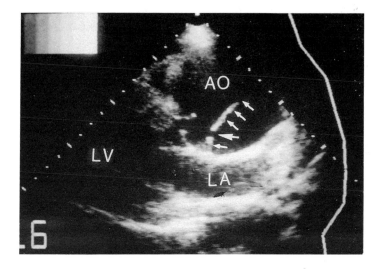

a) The slide shows a parasternal long axis view from a patient with an aortic dissection. Note the dilated (7 cm) ascending aorta with a posteriorly situated intimal flap (arrows).

Ao = Ascending aorta, LA = Left atrium, LV = Left ventricle.

The thoracic aorta is the commonest site for dissecting aneurysms. The dissection usually starts in the ascending aorta and extends to involve the arch, descending and abdominal aorta. Extension may thus result in limb ischaemia, spinal artery occlusion, mesenteric infarction and renal failure.

b) Dissecting aneurysms commonly occur in men aged between 40 and 70 years; predisposing factors include hypertension, coarctation of the aorta and Marfan's syndrome.

Tearing interscapular pain is the commonest presenting symptom with pain radiating into the neck and arms. Other presenting complaints include pleuritic chest pain, cardiac pain (as the dissection occludes a coronary ostium), syncope and dyspnoea. Clinical signs include an aortic diastolic murmur, a pericardial friction rub and a difference in blood pressure or radial pulse between the right and left arms.

The chest X-ray may show widening of the upper mediastinum but this is unreliable. The diagnosis, if suspected, should be confirmed using either echocardiography, CT scanning or angiography.

Immediate management of a thoracic aortic dissection involves pain relief and control of blood pressure followed by surgical repair of the aorta. Overall, 50% die within five days and 90% within six months.

a) What sign is present in slide A?
b) What sign is present in slide B? This patient also had a right ulnar nerve lesion and a left common peroneal nerve lesion.
c) What underlying disease do these patients have in common?

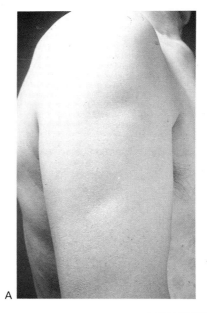

A

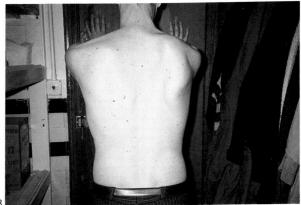

B

a) Diabetic lipoatrophy.
Diabetic lipodystrophy may take two forms:

1. Lipoatrophy as shown here is associated with injections of impure insulins; it is believed that in some way impurities lead to local lipolysis. Areas of lipodystrophy can be successfully treated by injecting pure insulin into the lesion, stimulating lipid synthesis.
2. Lipohypertrophy is the commonest variety in countries which use highly purified insulins and is due to repeated injections at the same site. It can be prevented by rotation of injection sites. Local lipid synthesis probably results from a high local concentration of insulin. Injection into an area of lipohypertrophy is associated with delayed absorption of insulin.

b) Winging of the scapula — lesion of the long thoracic nerve (nerve roots C5, 6, 7) resulting in weakness of serratus anterior, best demonstrated by resisted forward extension of the arm. The long thoracic nerve lesion is part of a mononeuritis multiplex.
Differential diagnosis of mononeuritis multiplex:

1. Diabetes mellitus
2. Sarcoidosis
3. Rheumatoid arthritis
4. Polyarteritis nodosa (Churg–Strauss syndrome)
5. Malignancy
6. Leprosy
7. AIDS.

c) Diabetes mellitus.
Diabetic neuropathy may take several forms:

1. Peripheral sensory glove and stocking neuropathy
2. Proximal motor neuropathy
3. Mononeuropathy/involvement of several peripheral nerves simultaneously can result in a mononeuritis multiplex picture
4. Autonomic neuropathy.

a) What is the radiological abnormality?
b) Give a differential diagnosis.

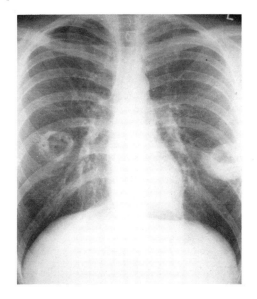

a) There are two well demarcated cavitating lesions present.
b) Differential diagnosis of cavitating nodules on a chest X-ray includes:

1. Abscesses
   — Post aspiration (especially in unconscious patients following anaesthesia, excess alcohol consumption, epileptic fit, etc)
   — Pneumonia, especially staphylococci or klebsiella
2. Neoplasm
   — primary or secondary tumours
3. Tuberculosis — particularly upper lobes, often associated with calcification
4. Pulmonary infarction — especially if caused by emboli from an infected valve (e.g. i.v. drug addicts) or venous lines (patients on chemotherapy or haemodialysis)
5. Rheumatoid nodules
6. Granulomas — Wegener's granulomatosis
7. Fungal infections — aspergilloma, histoplasmosis, coccidioidomycosis
8. Bullae — commonly thin walled
9. Pneumoconiosis or pulmonary fibrosis
10. Cystic fibrosis
11. Hydatid cysts.

Describe the radiological abnormality present. What is the diagnosis?

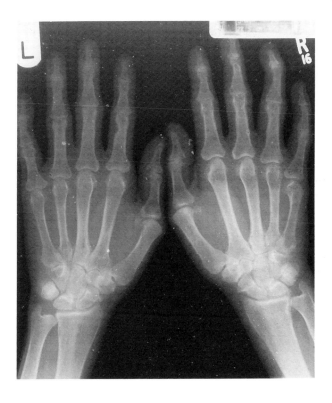

Hyperparathyroidism — the slide shows marked subperiosteal resorption of the phalanges. Evidence of subperiosteal resorption is often best seen on the radial side of the proximal and middle phalanges of the hand, the lateral ends of the clavicle and sites of muscle insertion, e.g. the ischial tuberosities. Other radiological signs of hyperparathyroidism include:

1. Resorption of the tufts of the terminal phalanges
2. Multiple osteolytic lesions in the skull (pepper pot skull)
3. Osteitis fibrosa cystica, often called 'brown tumours', which represent osteoclastic resorption and fibrosis; these may be seen in the long bones, ribs and phalanges.

Such radiological features are seen in both primary and secondary hyperparathyroidism. Secondary hyperparathyroidism is often accompanied by osteomalacia and the X-ray findings associated with vitamin D deficiency.

a) What clinical sign is shown?
b) This man presented with bilateral ptosis and diplopia. What is the likely diagnosis?

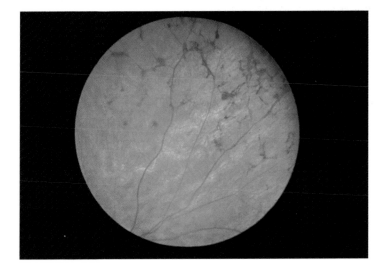

a) Retinitis pigmentation.
b) Kearns–Sayre syndrome.

The characteristic features of Kearns–Sayre syndrome are progressive external ophthalmoplegia with pigmentary retinopathy presenting before 20 years of age with one or more of the following:

1. Cardiac conduction defects
2. Ataxia
3. A high CSF protein.

Other recognized features include deafness, short stature, diabetes and hypoparathyroidism.
Deletions of mitochondrial DNA in muscle biopsies are seen in over 80% of such patients.

What is the diagnosis?

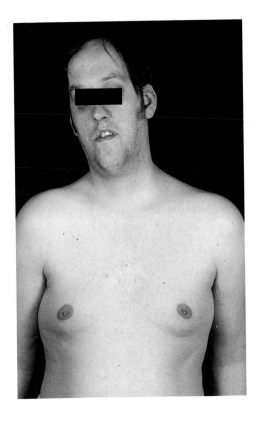

Dystrophia myotonica.

The typical facial appearances of frontal balding, expressionless forehead and ptosis is readily apparent.

Dystrophia myotonica is an autosomal dominant disorder that is recognized to demonstrate anticipation. This means that disease expression occurs earlier and more severely with successive generations. The genetic defect lies on chromosome 19 and it is presumed that the harmful gene product in some way damages normal tissues.

Clinical features include:

1. Wasting and weakness of the facial muscles, leading to bilateral ptosis and expressionless forehead; in the limbs, the forearm muscles are particularly affected
2. Frontal balding
3. Cataracts
4. Gonadal atrophy
5. Cardiomyopathy
6. Oesophageal dysmotility
7. Impaired pulmonary ventilation
8. Low IQ.

a) What is the clinical diagnosis?
b) What investigation has been performed and what does it show?

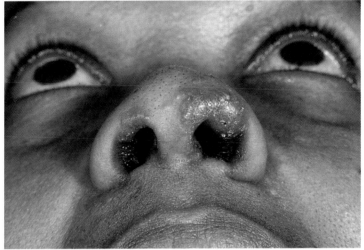

A

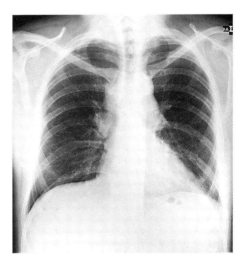

B

a) The typical red nodular lesions of lupus pernio are well seen. These chronic persistent disfiguring lesions are commoner in women and much more florid in blacks than whites. Lupus pernio is closely associated with sarcoidosis affecting the upper respiratory tract and overall is associated with the chronic fibrotic type of sarcoid. The cutaneous manifestations of sarcoidosis are many and varied and include:

1. Erythema nodosum
2. Papulonodular sarcoid — smooth red-brown lesions which can occur anywhere on the body
3. Annular sarcoid
4. Scar sarcoid.

b) The investigation was a PA chest x-ray, which demonstrated bilateral hilar lymphadenopathy. Although the diagnosis of sarcoid is established by demonstrating non-caseating granulomas from two sites, the clinical presentation of a young black woman with lupus pernio and bilateral hilar lymphadenopathy is typical of sarcoidosis. Other investigations which may be helpful are serum ACE levels (elevated in 70% of sarcoidosis patients), and gallium scans which demonstrate increased uptake in involved sites. Bronchoscopy and biopsy, and bronchoalveolar lavage are often performed as part of the diagnostic work up.

This 65-year-old Indian man presented with fever, night sweats and weight loss.
a) What abnormality was apparent over the left chest wall?
b) What is the likely diagnosis?

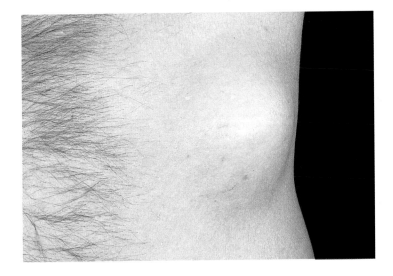

a) A large cold abscess is apparent.
b) Tuberculosis. The patient had previously been treated for pulmonary tuberculosis in India.

The abscess was aspirated and mycobacteria were visible on Ziehl–Neelsen staining. Chest X-ray showed extensive pleural calcification on the left consistent with previous pleural tuberculosis. The patient was commenced on triple therapy awaiting mycobacteria sensitivity studies, and surgical decortication was performed.

This patient has been treated for Wilson's disease for 10 years. What complication has occurred?

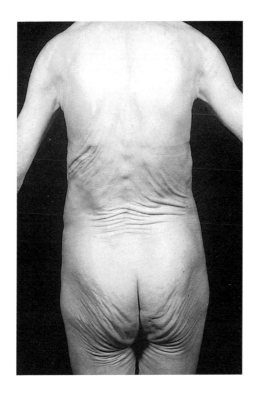

Cutis laxa.

This is a recognized side effect of treatment with high dose penicillamine. Penicillamine is the first line drug for Wilson's disease, and acts by chelating copper. High dosages, up to 2g a day, are used at first and the dose then titrated down as body copper stores are depleted. Adverse side effects of penicillamine are common and include rash, thrombocytopenia, granulocytopenia, lymphadenopathy and proteinuria (nephrotic syndrome in up to 8% of patients). Autoimmune diseases such as Goodpasture's syndrome and SLE have also been reported. Penicillamine has been used with some success in the treatment of diffuse systemic sclerosis to prevent skin thickening. Not surprisingly, some patients given high dosages develop lax skin due to inhibition of cross linking of collagen and elastin in the subcutaneous tissues.

Index

NB: Numbers in the index refer to
questions not pages.

6554 17178